The Complete Wellness Handbook:

Holistic Guide of Natural Protocols for Common Health Issues - Wellness Book

Contents

- Introduction 5
  - Welcome to Holistic Wellness 5
  - The Philosophy of Natural Healing 5
  - How to Use This Book 7
- Understanding Holistic Protocols 10
  - What is Holistic Medicine? 10
  - The Role of Herbal Remedies 11
  - Integrating Nutrition, Exercise, and Lifestyle Changes 14
- Herbal Protocols for Common Health Issues 17
  - Chronic Pain Management 17
  - Inflammatory Bowel Disease (IBD) 20
  - Brain and Nerve Health 23
  - Gastroesophageal Reflux Disease (GERD) and Acid Reflux 27
  - Prostate Health 31
  - Lung Health and Chronic Obstructive Pulmonary Disease (COPD) 34
  - Parkinson's Disease 39
  - Type-2 Diabetes 43
  - Leaky Gut, Gastritis, and Irritable Bowel Syndrome (IBS) 47
  - Lupus 53
  - Lyme Disease 56
  - Multiple Sclerosis 60
  - Adrenal Fatigue 64
  - Parasites 67
  - Candida Overgrowth 71
  - Anti-Aging Strategies 74
  - Flu, Viral, and Immune System Support 78
  - Bacterial Infections 82
  - Psoriasis and Eczema 86
  - Vertigo and Tinnitus 90
  - Thyroid Health 93
  - Allergies 97

- Alzheimer's and Dementia 101
- Heart Health 105
- Menopause Support 109
- Men's Sexual Health 113
- Sleep Disorders 117
- Weight Loss 120

Creating Your Personalized Wellness Plan 125
- Assessing Your Health Needs 125
- Choosing the Right Protocols 128
- Tracking Your Progress 130

Herbal Remedies and Supplements 133
- Essential Herbs for Wellness 133
- How to Make Herbal Remedies 136
- Supplement Recommendations 139

Nutrition for Optimal Health 144
- Anti-Inflammatory Diet 144
- Superfoods for Healing 146

Lifestyle and Exercise 149
- Stress Reduction Techniques 149
- Exercise Routines for Different Health Conditions 152
- The Importance of Sleep 157

Detoxification and Cleansing 161
- Safe Detox Practices 161
- Daily Detox Tips 163

Mind-Body Connection 167
- The Role of Mindfulness and Meditation 167
- Yoga and Stretching Exercises 170
- Emotional Wellness 174

Conclusion 178

Introduction

Welcome to Holistic Wellness

Welcome to **"The Complete Wellness Handbook: Holistic Guide of Natural Protocols for Common Health Issues."** This book is your comprehensive guide to embracing a holistic approach to health and wellness, designed to empower you with the knowledge and tools needed to achieve optimal well-being.

In today's fast-paced world, many of us have become reliant on quick fixes and symptom-focused treatments that often fail to address the root causes of our health issues. Holistic wellness, however, offers a different path—one that looks at the body as a whole and seeks to restore balance through natural and integrative methods.

This book is based on the principle that true health encompasses the harmony of our physical, emotional, and spiritual selves. By exploring the interconnectedness of these aspects, we can unlock the body's innate ability to heal and thrive. Through detailed protocols, practical advice, and a wealth of information, this handbook aims to guide you on your journey to holistic wellness.

You will find a wide range of topics covered in this book, from chronic pain management to digestive health, from stress reduction to immune support. Each section is thoughtfully crafted to provide you with step-by-step guidance on using herbal remedies, nutritional strategies, lifestyle modifications, and mind-body practices to achieve lasting health benefits.

Whether you are new to holistic health or have been on this journey for some time, **"The Complete Wellness Handbook"** offers valuable insights and actionable steps to help you take control of your health naturally. Let this book be your companion as you navigate the path to a healthier, more balanced, and fulfilling life.

Welcome to a new chapter of wellness, where natural protocols and holistic practices pave the way to your best self.

The Philosophy of Natural Healing

At the heart of **"The Complete Wellness Handbook"** lies the philosophy of natural healing—a belief system that recognizes the body's inherent capacity to heal itself when given the proper support. This approach transcends merely addressing symptoms, focusing instead on understanding and correcting the underlying imbalances that cause illness.

Natural healing is rooted in the idea that the body, mind, and spirit are interconnected. When one aspect of our being is out of balance, it can affect our overall health. Holistic wellness aims to restore harmony across all these dimensions by employing a wide array of natural therapies and lifestyle practices.

Core Principles of Natural Healing

1. **Treat the Root Cause**: Unlike conventional medicine, which often focuses on symptom management, natural healing seeks to identify and address the root causes of health issues. By understanding the underlying imbalances, we can develop strategies that promote long-term health and prevent recurrence.

2. **Support the Whole Person**: Holistic wellness considers the physical, emotional, mental, and spiritual aspects of health. Treatments and protocols are designed to support the whole person, recognizing that true healing involves more than just the physical body.

3. **Use Natural Therapies**: Natural healing relies on a variety of therapies that are derived from nature. This includes herbal remedies, nutrition, exercise, detoxification, and mind-body practices. These therapies work synergistically to enhance the body's natural healing processes.

4. **Promote Self-Care and Empowerment**: A key component of natural healing is empowering individuals to take an active role in their health. By providing the knowledge and tools necessary for self-care, this approach encourages personal responsibility and informed decision-making.

5. **Preventive Focus**: Natural healing emphasizes prevention as much as treatment. By maintaining a balanced lifestyle, managing stress, and using natural remedies proactively, we can prevent many health issues from developing in the first place.

The Role of Herbal Remedies

Herbal medicine is a cornerstone of natural healing. Plants have been used for centuries across various cultures for their medicinal properties. Modern research continues to validate the efficacy of many herbs in treating a wide range of health conditions. By incorporating herbal remedies into your wellness plan, you can benefit from their powerful healing properties.

Integrating Nutrition, Exercise, and Lifestyle Changes

Nutrition plays a vital role in natural healing. An anti-inflammatory diet rich in whole foods, vitamins, and minerals supports overall health and helps mitigate chronic conditions. Regular physical activity, tailored to individual needs, strengthens the body and mind, while lifestyle changes, such as stress management and adequate sleep, further enhance wellness.

The Mind-Body Connection

The mind and body are deeply interconnected, and emotional well-being is essential to physical health. Practices such as mindfulness, meditation, and yoga can reduce stress, improve mental clarity, and promote emotional balance. Addressing mental and emotional health is crucial for achieving holistic wellness.

Embracing Natural Healing

Embracing the philosophy of natural healing means committing to a journey of self-discovery and continuous improvement. It involves being open to learning, trying new practices, and making gradual, sustainable changes. By adopting this holistic approach, you are not just treating illnesses but fostering a lifestyle that promotes long-term health and vitality.

Welcome to the world of natural healing. May this book serve as a guiding light on your path to holistic wellness.

How to Use This Book

Welcome to **"The Complete Wellness Handbook: Holistic Guide of Natural Protocols for Common Health Issues."** This book is designed to be a comprehensive resource for anyone seeking to enhance their health through natural and holistic methods. To get the most out of this book, here are some guidelines on how to navigate and utilize the information presented:

Understanding the Structure

This book is divided into several key sections, each focused on different aspects of holistic wellness:

1. **Introduction**: Provides an overview of holistic wellness and the philosophy of natural healing.

2. **Understanding Holistic Protocols**: Explains the principles behind holistic medicine and the role of various natural therapies.

3. **Herbal Protocols for Common Health Issues**: Details specific protocols for a wide range of health conditions, including herbal remedies, dietary recommendations, and lifestyle changes.

4. **Creating Your Personalized Wellness Plan**: Guides you through assessing your health needs and developing a tailored wellness plan.

5. **Herbal Remedies and Supplements**: Offers information on essential herbs and supplements, including preparation and usage.

6. **Nutrition for Optimal Health**: Covers dietary strategies, superfoods, and recipes to support health and healing.

7. **Lifestyle and Exercise**: Provides tips on stress reduction, exercise routines, and the importance of sleep.
8. **Detoxification and Cleansing**: Discusses safe detox practices and daily detox tips.
9. **Mind-Body Connection**: Explores mindfulness, meditation, yoga, and emotional wellness practices.
10. **Resources and References**: Lists additional resources, recommended readings, and trusted suppliers.
11. **Conclusion**: Summarizes key points and offers long-term wellness strategies.

Navigating the Protocols

Each health issue in the **"Herbal Protocols for Common Health Issues"** section is presented with a detailed protocol that includes:

- **Description of the Condition**: An overview of the health issue, including symptoms and common causes.
- **Herbal Remedies**: Specific herbs that can help address the condition, with instructions on how to use them.
- **Dietary Recommendations**: Foods that support healing and those to avoid.
- **Lifestyle Modifications**: Exercises, stretches, and other lifestyle changes that can benefit your condition.
- **Mind-Body Practices**: Techniques such as meditation, breathing exercises, and yoga that can aid in recovery.
- **Additional Tips**: Other useful practices, such as detoxification methods or supplements, that can enhance your healing process.

Creating Your Personalized Wellness Plan

In the **"Creating Your Personalized Wellness Plan"** section, you'll find guidance on:

- **Assessing Your Health Needs**: Tools and strategies for evaluating your current health status.
- **Choosing the Right Protocols**: How to select the most appropriate protocols based on your individual needs.
- **Tracking Your Progress**: Methods for monitoring your progress and making adjustments as needed.

Utilizing the Herbal Remedies and Supplements

The **"Herbal Remedies and Supplements"** section provides:

- **Essential Herbs**: A list of key herbs, their benefits, and how to use them.
- **Preparation Methods**: Instructions for making teas, tinctures, salves, and other herbal preparations.
- **Supplement Recommendations**: Guidance on choosing and using supplements to support your health.

Incorporating Nutrition, Lifestyle, and Mind-Body Practices

The sections on **Nutrition for Optimal Health**, **Lifestyle and Exercise**, and **Mind-Body Connection** offer practical advice on:

- **Healthy Eating**: Anti-inflammatory diets, superfoods, and healing recipes.
- **Exercise Routines**: Physical activities tailored to different health conditions.
- **Stress Management**: Techniques to reduce stress and improve emotional well-being.

Using the Resources and References

The **Resources and References** section includes:

- **Recommended Reading**: Books and articles for further learning.
- **Herbal Suppliers and Tools**: Trusted sources for purchasing herbs and supplies.
- **Index**: An alphabetical listing of topics covered in the book for quick reference.

Making the Most of This Book

- **Start with the Basics**: Begin by reading the introductory sections to build a foundation of understanding about holistic wellness and natural healing.
- **Focus on Your Needs**: Identify the health issues that are most relevant to you and explore the corresponding protocols in detail.
- **Take Notes**: Keep a journal to record your observations, progress, and any adjustments you make to your wellness plan.
- **Be Patient and Consistent**: Holistic healing is a gradual process. Consistency and patience are key to achieving lasting results.
- **Seek Professional Guidance**: While this book provides comprehensive information, consulting with a healthcare professional, especially one experienced in holistic medicine, can offer additional support and personalized advice.

By following these guidelines, you can effectively utilize **"The Complete Wellness Handbook"** to enhance your health and well-being through natural and holistic methods. Welcome to a journey of empowerment and healing.

Understanding Holistic Protocols

What is Holistic Medicine?

Holistic medicine is a comprehensive approach to health care that emphasizes treating the whole person—mind, body, and spirit—rather than just focusing on specific symptoms or diseases. This philosophy of care recognizes the interconnectedness of all aspects of an individual's life and seeks to promote overall well-being by addressing the root causes of illness.

The Core Principles of Holistic Medicine

1. **Whole-Person Care**: Holistic medicine views the person as an integrated whole, where physical health is inseparable from emotional, mental, and spiritual well-being. Treatment plans are designed to support all aspects of an individual's life.

2. **Prevention and Wellness**: Instead of waiting for illness to occur, holistic medicine emphasizes prevention and the maintenance of good health. This includes promoting healthy lifestyle choices, balanced nutrition, regular exercise, stress management, and the cultivation of positive relationships.

3. **Personalized Treatment**: Each individual is unique, and holistic medicine tailors treatments to meet the specific needs, circumstances, and goals of the patient. This personalized approach ensures that care is relevant and effective.

4. **Empowerment and Self-Care**: Holistic medicine encourages patients to take an active role in their own health. By educating individuals on the importance of self-care practices, holistic medicine empowers them to make informed decisions that enhance their well-being.

5. **Natural and Integrative Therapies**: Holistic medicine often incorporates natural therapies, such as herbal remedies, nutrition, acupuncture, yoga, meditation, and chiropractic care. These therapies can be used alongside conventional medicine, creating an integrative approach that leverages the strengths of both traditional and alternative treatments.

How Holistic Medicine Differs from Conventional Medicine

While conventional medicine typically focuses on diagnosing and treating specific diseases with pharmaceuticals or surgery, holistic medicine looks at the broader context of an individual's life. Here are some key differences:

- **Focus on Root Causes**: Holistic practitioners aim to identify and address the root causes of illness, not just the symptoms. For example, instead of prescribing medication for chronic headaches, a holistic approach might explore dietary factors, stress levels, posture, or emotional well-being as potential contributors.

- **Use of Natural Remedies**: Holistic medicine often favors natural remedies, such as herbs, dietary changes, and lifestyle modifications, over synthetic drugs. These remedies work to support the body's natural healing processes and often have fewer side effects.

- **Mind-Body-Spirit Connection**: Holistic medicine strongly emphasizes the connection between mind, body, and spirit. Practices such as meditation, mindfulness, and energy healing are commonly used to promote overall well-being and address the emotional or spiritual dimensions of health.

Benefits of Holistic Medicine

- **Comprehensive Care**: By treating the whole person, holistic medicine addresses the complexities of human health, leading to more comprehensive care.

- **Personalized Attention**: Holistic practitioners spend time understanding their patients' lifestyles, beliefs, and health goals, providing care that is uniquely tailored to each individual.

- **Focus on Prevention**: The emphasis on prevention and self-care helps individuals maintain health and reduce the risk of chronic diseases.

- **Complementary to Conventional Medicine**: Holistic medicine can be used alongside conventional treatments, offering a well-rounded approach to health care.

The Role of the Patient in Holistic Medicine

In holistic medicine, the patient is not a passive recipient of care but an active participant in the healing process. This approach encourages individuals to be mindful of their health, make informed choices, and engage in practices that promote their overall well-being. By taking responsibility for their health, patients can achieve better outcomes and enjoy a higher quality of life.

Holistic medicine is more than just a method of treatment; it is a philosophy of living that promotes balance, harmony, and wellness in all areas of life. As you explore the protocols and practices in this book, keep in mind the holistic principles of treating the whole person and addressing the root causes of illness. This approach will guide you toward a healthier, more fulfilling life.

The Role of Herbal Remedies

Herbal remedies play a central role in holistic medicine, offering a natural and time-honored approach to healing and maintaining health. For thousands of years, cultures around the world have relied on the medicinal properties of plants to treat a wide array of ailments, and modern science continues to validate the efficacy of many of these traditional remedies.

What Are Herbal Remedies?

Herbal remedies are medicines made from plants or plant extracts. These remedies can include various parts of a plant—such as the leaves, flowers, roots, seeds, or bark—and are often used in the form of teas, tinctures, capsules, powders, or topical applications. The active compounds in these plants work to promote healing, restore balance, and support the body's natural functions.

How Herbal Remedies Support Healing

1. **Addressing the Root Cause of Illness**: Unlike conventional medicines that often focus on alleviating symptoms, herbal remedies are typically used to address the underlying causes of health issues. For example, rather than just reducing inflammation, an herbal remedy might also strengthen the immune system, improve digestion, or support detoxification processes, depending on the root cause of the inflammation.

2. **Supporting the Body's Natural Healing Processes**: Herbal remedies are designed to enhance the body's innate ability to heal itself. They provide the nutrients and compounds necessary for repairing tissues, fighting infections, and restoring balance to bodily systems.

3. **Balancing the Body's Systems**: Many herbs are adaptogens, meaning they help the body adapt to stress and maintain equilibrium. Adaptogenic herbs, such as ashwagandha, rhodiola, and holy basil, support the adrenal glands and help regulate hormones, improving the body's resilience to stress and illness.

4. **Preventing Disease**: Herbal remedies can also be used proactively to prevent illness. For instance, herbs like echinacea and elderberry are known for their immune-boosting properties, helping to ward off colds and flu. Regular use of certain herbs can fortify the body against environmental toxins, pathogens, and stressors.

5. **Reducing Side Effects**: One of the advantages of herbal remedies is that they often have fewer side effects compared to synthetic drugs. When used correctly, herbs can provide effective treatment with a lower risk of adverse reactions, making them a safer option for long-term use.

Common Forms of Herbal Remedies

- **Teas and Infusions**: Herbal teas are one of the simplest and most traditional ways to use herbs. By steeping herbs in hot water, you can extract their beneficial compounds. Teas are commonly used for digestive issues, relaxation, and overall health maintenance.

- **Tinctures and Extracts**: Tinctures are concentrated liquid extracts made by soaking herbs in alcohol or glycerin. They are potent and easily absorbed by the body, making them an effective form of herbal medicine.
- **Capsules and Tablets**: These are convenient forms of herbal remedies that allow for precise dosing. They are ideal for individuals who need specific amounts of an herb and prefer not to taste the herbs.
- **Topical Applications**: Herbal remedies can also be applied externally in the form of salves, ointments, and poultices. These are commonly used for skin conditions, wounds, and muscle pain.
- **Essential Oils**: Distilled from plants, essential oils are highly concentrated and used in aromatherapy, massage, and skin care. They have various therapeutic properties, including anti-inflammatory, antiseptic, and calming effects.

Integrating Herbal Remedies into Holistic Protocols

Herbal remedies are a key component of holistic protocols, which are comprehensive treatment plans designed to address specific health issues. In these protocols, herbs are often combined with other natural therapies, such as nutrition, exercise, and stress management, to create a synergistic effect that enhances healing.

For example:

- **In a protocol for managing anxiety**, calming herbs like lavender, valerian, and chamomile might be paired with mindfulness practices, a balanced diet, and regular physical activity to provide comprehensive support.
- **In a protocol for digestive health**, herbs like ginger, peppermint, and licorice root could be combined with dietary changes, probiotic supplements, and stress reduction techniques to restore gut balance and improve digestion.

Choosing and Using Herbal Remedies Safely

While herbal remedies are generally safe, it is important to use them correctly to avoid potential interactions or side effects. Here are some guidelines for safe use:

- **Consult a Professional**: If you are new to herbal medicine or have existing health conditions, it's advisable to consult with a healthcare provider, especially one knowledgeable in herbal medicine, before starting any new herbal regimen.
- **Follow Dosage Instructions**: Always adhere to recommended dosages and be mindful of how your body responds. More is not always better with herbs, and excessive use can lead to unwanted effects.

- **Consider Quality and Source**: Use high-quality, organic herbs from reputable sources to ensure potency and safety. Herbs should be free from contaminants and pesticides.

Embracing the Healing Power of Herbs

Incorporating herbal remedies into your wellness routine is a powerful way to take control of your health. Whether you're looking to address a specific health issue, prevent illness, or simply maintain overall well-being, herbs offer a natural and effective solution. As you explore the protocols in this book, you'll discover the many ways in which herbal remedies can support your journey toward holistic health.

Integrating Nutrition, Exercise, and Lifestyle Changes

In holistic medicine, the integration of nutrition, exercise, and lifestyle changes is essential for achieving and maintaining optimal health. These foundational elements work synergistically with herbal remedies and other natural therapies to support the body's natural healing processes, prevent disease, and promote overall well-being.

The Power of Nutrition

Nutrition is a cornerstone of holistic health, as what you eat directly impacts your body's ability to function, heal, and thrive. A balanced, nutrient-rich diet can prevent many chronic diseases, boost energy levels, enhance mental clarity, and support a strong immune system.

Key Principles of Holistic Nutrition:

1. **Whole Foods**: Emphasize whole, unprocessed foods such as fruits, vegetables, whole grains, nuts, seeds, and lean proteins. These foods provide essential nutrients, fiber, and antioxidants that support overall health.

2. **Anti-Inflammatory Diet**: Chronic inflammation is at the root of many health issues. A diet rich in anti-inflammatory foods—like leafy greens, berries, fatty fish, turmeric, and ginger—can help reduce inflammation and promote healing.

3. **Balanced Macronutrients**: Ensure a balance of carbohydrates, proteins, and fats in your diet. Each macronutrient plays a vital role in energy production, muscle repair, and hormone regulation.

4. **Superfoods**: Incorporate nutrient-dense superfoods such as chia seeds, spirulina, blueberries, and avocados to boost your intake of vitamins, minerals, and antioxidants.

5. **Hydration**: Adequate water intake is crucial for maintaining bodily functions, supporting detoxification, and promoting healthy skin and digestion.

6. **Mindful Eating**: Practice mindful eating by paying attention to hunger and fullness cues, chewing food thoroughly, and savoring the flavors and textures of your meals. This can improve digestion and foster a healthy relationship with food.

The Role of Exercise

Regular physical activity is vital for maintaining physical, mental, and emotional health. Exercise helps to strengthen the cardiovascular system, build and maintain muscle mass, support joint health, and improve mood through the release of endorphins.

Incorporating Exercise into Holistic Wellness:

1. **Variety**: Incorporate a variety of exercises to address different aspects of fitness. This includes cardiovascular exercises like walking, running, or cycling; strength training; flexibility exercises such as yoga or Pilates; and balance and coordination activities.

2. **Consistency**: Regularity is key. Aim for at least 150 minutes of moderate-intensity aerobic activity per week, along with muscle-strengthening activities on two or more days per week.

3. **Adaptation**: Choose exercises that suit your current fitness level and health status. As your fitness improves, gradually increase the intensity and duration of your workouts.

4. **Mind-Body Connection**: Engage in exercises that also promote mental well-being, such as yoga, Tai Chi, or Qigong. These practices integrate movement with breath control and meditation, fostering a strong connection between mind and body.

5. **Recovery**: Allow time for rest and recovery between intense workouts to prevent injury and support muscle repair and growth.

Lifestyle Changes for Holistic Health

Beyond nutrition and exercise, certain lifestyle changes are crucial for achieving and maintaining holistic health. These changes help reduce stress, improve mental clarity, and promote overall well-being.

Essential Lifestyle Changes:

1. **Stress Management**: Chronic stress can have detrimental effects on health, leading to issues like hypertension, anxiety, and digestive disorders. Incorporate stress-reducing practices such as meditation, deep breathing exercises, journaling, or spending time in nature to help manage stress effectively.

2. **Sleep Hygiene**: Quality sleep is essential for physical and mental recovery. Establish a regular sleep routine, create a restful environment, and avoid stimulants like caffeine close to bedtime to improve sleep quality.

3. **Detoxification**: Support your body's natural detoxification processes by consuming a diet rich in fiber, drinking plenty of water, and incorporating detoxifying herbs like dandelion and milk thistle. Regularly sweating through exercise or sauna use can also aid in detoxification.

4. **Healthy Relationships**: Foster positive relationships and a supportive social network. Emotional well-being is closely linked to the quality of your relationships, and healthy connections can provide a sense of belonging, reduce stress, and improve overall happiness.

5. **Environmental Awareness**: Be mindful of your environment, including the quality of the air you breathe, the water you drink, and the products you use on your body and in your home. Reducing exposure to toxins and pollutants is important for maintaining health.

6. **Mindful Living**: Cultivate mindfulness in your daily life. This involves being present in the moment, practicing gratitude, and approaching life's challenges with a positive and balanced mindset.

Creating a Holistic Wellness Plan

To effectively integrate nutrition, exercise, and lifestyle changes into your holistic wellness plan, follow these steps:

1. **Assess Your Current Habits**: Take an honest look at your current diet, exercise routine, and lifestyle habits. Identify areas that need improvement and set realistic, achievable goals.

2. **Start Small**: Make gradual changes rather than attempting a complete overhaul. Small, consistent steps lead to sustainable habits.

3. **Personalize Your Approach**: Tailor your plan to your unique needs, preferences, and health goals. What works for one person may not work for another, so it's important to find what suits you best.

4. **Track Your Progress**: Keep a journal or use a health app to track your progress, noting any improvements in your physical and mental well-being.

5. **Stay Flexible**: Be open to adjusting your plan as needed. Life changes, and your wellness plan should evolve with you.

Conclusion

Integrating nutrition, exercise, and lifestyle changes is essential for achieving holistic health. By adopting a balanced diet, engaging in regular physical activity, and making mindful lifestyle choices, you can create a strong foundation for lasting wellness. These practices not only support physical health but also contribute to emotional and mental well-being, helping you lead a vibrant and fulfilling life.

Herbal Protocols for Common Health Issues

Chronic Pain Management

Chronic pain can be debilitating and affects millions of people worldwide. Managing chronic pain effectively often requires a multifaceted approach that includes not only addressing the pain itself but also the underlying causes. This protocol focuses on natural strategies, including the use of herbal remedies, nutrition, exercise, and lifestyle changes to help manage and reduce chronic pain.

Key Herbs for Chronic Pain Management

1. **Turmeric (Curcuma longa)**:
    - **Properties**: Anti-inflammatory, antioxidant
    - **Usage**: Turmeric contains curcumin, a compound known for its strong anti-inflammatory effects. It can be taken as a supplement, added to foods, or consumed as a tea.

2. **Ginger (Zingiber officinale)**:
    - **Properties**: Anti-inflammatory, analgesic
    - **Usage**: Ginger helps reduce inflammation and pain, particularly in conditions like arthritis. It can be taken as a tea, added to meals, or used as a supplement.

3. **Devil's Claw (Harpagophytum procumbens)**:
    - **Properties**: Anti-inflammatory, analgesic
    - **Usage**: Commonly used for back pain, arthritis, and muscle pain, Devil's Claw can be taken in capsule form or as a tincture.

4. **White Willow Bark (Salix alba)**:
    - **Properties**: Analgesic, anti-inflammatory
    - **Usage**: Often referred to as "nature's aspirin," white willow bark is effective in reducing pain and inflammation. It can be used as a tea, tincture, or supplement.

5. **Boswellia (Boswellia serrata)**:
    - **Properties**: Anti-inflammatory

- **Usage**: Boswellia is particularly effective for inflammatory conditions such as arthritis. It can be taken as a capsule or tincture.

Dietary Recommendations

1. **Anti-Inflammatory Diet**:
    - Focus on foods that reduce inflammation, such as:
        - **Fatty Fish** (e.g., salmon, mackerel): High in omega-3 fatty acids, which are known for their anti-inflammatory properties.
        - **Leafy Greens** (e.g., spinach, kale): Rich in antioxidants and vitamins that reduce inflammation.
        - **Berries** (e.g., blueberries, strawberries): Packed with antioxidants like anthocyanins that help lower inflammation.
        - **Nuts and Seeds** (e.g., almonds, chia seeds): Provide healthy fats and antioxidants.

2. **Avoid Inflammatory Foods**:
    - Reduce or eliminate foods that can increase inflammation and pain, such as:
        - **Processed Foods**: High in unhealthy fats, sugars, and preservatives.
        - **Refined Carbohydrates**: Such as white bread, pastries, and sugary snacks.
        - **Red Meat**: Particularly processed and high-fat cuts.

3. **Hydration**:
    - Drink plenty of water to stay hydrated, which helps flush out toxins that may contribute to inflammation and pain.

Exercise and Physical Activity

1. **Low-Impact Exercises**:
    - **Swimming**: Offers a full-body workout without putting strain on the joints.
    - **Yoga**: Improves flexibility, strength, and mental focus, while reducing stress.
    - **Walking**: Regular walking can improve circulation, reduce stiffness, and boost overall mood.

2. **Stretching**:

- Regular stretching helps maintain flexibility and reduces muscle tightness that can exacerbate pain. Focus on gentle, slow stretches, especially for the affected areas.

3. **Strength Training**:
    - Building muscle strength, particularly in the core and surrounding muscles, can reduce the burden on joints and alleviate pain. Use light weights or resistance bands and focus on proper form.

Lifestyle Changes

1. **Stress Management**:
    - **Meditation**: Regular practice can help reduce the perception of pain by promoting relaxation and reducing stress.
    - **Deep Breathing Exercises**: Helps to calm the nervous system and reduce pain perception.
    - **Journaling**: Writing about your pain and emotions can help process and manage chronic pain more effectively.

2. **Sleep Hygiene**:
    - Adequate and restful sleep is crucial for pain management. Create a calming bedtime routine, avoid screens before bed, and ensure your sleeping environment is comfortable and quiet.

3. **Posture and Ergonomics**:
    - Proper posture, especially during activities like sitting at a desk or lifting objects, can significantly reduce strain on your body and minimize pain. Consider using ergonomic chairs and desks, and pay attention to body mechanics.

4. **Mind-Body Practices**:
    - **Tai Chi**: This gentle martial art can improve balance, flexibility, and pain management.
    - **Acupuncture**: Stimulates specific points on the body, which can help manage pain by promoting the release of endorphins and improving energy flow.

Additional Therapies

1. **Acupuncture**:
    - Effective for pain relief, particularly for chronic conditions like back pain, arthritis, and migraines.

2. **Massage Therapy**:
   - Helps to relax tight muscles, improve circulation, and reduce pain.
3. **Heat and Cold Therapy**:
   - Use heat to relax and loosen tissues and to stimulate blood flow to the area. Cold therapy can reduce inflammation and numb the pain.

Conclusion

Chronic pain management requires a holistic approach that includes the use of herbal remedies, proper nutrition, regular exercise, and key lifestyle changes. By addressing the root causes of pain and integrating these natural strategies into your daily routine, you can improve your quality of life and reduce your dependence on conventional pain medications. Always consult with a healthcare provider before starting any new treatment plan, especially if you have a pre-existing condition or are taking other medications.

Inflammatory Bowel Disease (IBD)

Inflammatory Bowel Disease (IBD) is a term primarily used to describe two chronic conditions, Crohn's disease and ulcerative colitis, that involve inflammation of the digestive tract. Managing IBD effectively requires a combination of dietary adjustments, herbal remedies, and lifestyle modifications to reduce inflammation, promote healing, and maintain remission.

Key Herbs for IBD Management

1. **Slippery Elm (Ulmus rubra)**:
   - **Properties**: Demulcent, anti-inflammatory, soothing to the digestive tract.
   - **Usage**: Slippery Elm can be taken as a powder mixed with water or as a tea to soothe the lining of the digestive tract and reduce irritation.
2. **Marshmallow Root (Althaea officinalis)**:
   - **Properties**: Demulcent, anti-inflammatory, protective of mucous membranes.
   - **Usage**: Marshmallow root can be consumed as a tea or tincture to coat the digestive tract and reduce inflammation.
3. **Aloe Vera (Aloe barbadensis miller)**:
   - **Properties**: Anti-inflammatory, soothing, promotes healing.
   - **Usage**: Aloe Vera juice can be taken internally to soothe the digestive tract and reduce inflammation.

4. **Boswellia (Boswellia serrata)**:
   - **Properties**: Anti-inflammatory, particularly useful for reducing inflammation in the digestive tract.
   - **Usage**: Boswellia can be taken as a capsule or tincture to help manage inflammation associated with IBD.

5. **Turmeric (Curcuma longa)**:
   - **Properties**: Anti-inflammatory, antioxidant.
   - **Usage**: Turmeric, particularly its active compound curcumin, can be taken as a supplement or added to foods to reduce inflammation in the gut.

Dietary Recommendations

1. **Low-Residue Diet**:
   - **Purpose**: Reduces the frequency and volume of bowel movements by minimizing the amount of undigested material passing through the intestines.
   - **Includes**:
     - **Refined grains**: White bread, white rice, and pasta.
     - **Cooked vegetables**: Without skins or seeds.
     - **Lean proteins**: Skinless poultry, fish, eggs.
   - **Avoid**: High-fiber foods such as raw vegetables, nuts, seeds, and whole grains during flare-ups.

2. **Anti-Inflammatory Foods**:
   - **Emphasize**: Foods rich in omega-3 fatty acids, like fatty fish (salmon, mackerel) and flaxseeds, as well as antioxidant-rich fruits like blueberries and anti-inflammatory spices like ginger and turmeric.

3. **Probiotic-Rich Foods**:
   - **Purpose**: To restore and maintain a healthy gut flora, which can be disrupted in IBD.
   - **Include**: Yogurt with live cultures, kefir, sauerkraut, kimchi, and other fermented foods.

4. **Hydration**:
   - **Importance**: Staying well-hydrated is crucial, especially during flare-ups when diarrhea is common. Drink plenty of water, herbal teas, and broths.

5. **Food Sensitivities**:
    - **Approach**: Identify and avoid specific food triggers that may exacerbate symptoms. Common triggers include dairy, gluten, and certain carbohydrates.

Exercise and Physical Activity

1. **Gentle Exercises**:
    - **Walking**: Regular, moderate walking can help improve digestion and reduce stress.
    - **Yoga**: Gentle yoga poses can aid in digestion, reduce stress, and enhance overall well-being.
    - **Tai Chi**: This slow, meditative form of exercise can help improve balance and reduce stress, which can be beneficial for managing IBD symptoms.

2. **Stretching**:
    - Gentle stretching can help alleviate abdominal discomfort and improve circulation, which supports overall digestive health.

Lifestyle Changes

1. **Stress Management**:
    - **Meditation**: Regular meditation can help reduce stress, which is a known trigger for IBD flare-ups.
    - **Deep Breathing**: Practicing deep breathing exercises can help calm the nervous system and reduce stress-related symptoms.
    - **Journaling**: Keeping a journal can help you track triggers and emotional responses that might exacerbate IBD symptoms.

2. **Sleep Hygiene**:
    - **Importance**: Adequate sleep is essential for healing and reducing inflammation. Aim for 7-9 hours of restful sleep each night.
    - **Tips**: Establish a regular sleep schedule, create a calming bedtime routine, and avoid screens before bed.

3. **Mindful Eating**:
    - **Practice**: Eat slowly, chew thoroughly, and focus on your food without distractions. Mindful eating can improve digestion and reduce symptoms.

4. **Environmental Awareness**:

- **Minimize Exposure**: Avoid exposure to environmental toxins, as they can exacerbate inflammation and IBD symptoms. This includes avoiding processed foods, artificial additives, and unnecessary medications when possible.

Additional Therapies

1. **Probiotics**:
   - **Usage**: Taking a high-quality probiotic supplement can help restore and maintain a healthy balance of gut bacteria, which is often disrupted in IBD.

2. **Digestive Enzymes**:
   - **Usage**: Supplementing with digestive enzymes can help improve nutrient absorption and reduce digestive discomfort.

3. **Acupuncture**:
   - **Benefits**: Acupuncture can help manage pain and stress, which can contribute to flare-ups in IBD.

4. **Heat Therapy**:
   - **Usage**: Applying a warm compress to the abdomen can help relieve cramping and discomfort during flare-ups.

Conclusion

Managing Inflammatory Bowel Disease requires a comprehensive approach that includes herbal remedies, dietary changes, gentle exercise, and stress management. By addressing the root causes of inflammation and promoting a healthy gut environment, this protocol aims to reduce the frequency and severity of IBD flare-ups, improve overall digestive health, and enhance quality of life. Always consult with a healthcare provider before starting any new treatment plan, especially if you have a chronic condition or are taking other medications.

Brain and Nerve Health

Maintaining brain and nerve health is crucial for cognitive function, memory, mood stability, and overall neurological well-being. This protocol focuses on natural strategies, including herbal remedies, nutrition, exercise, and lifestyle changes, to support and enhance brain and nerve health. The goal is to protect against neurodegenerative diseases, reduce cognitive decline, and promote mental clarity.

Key Herbs for Brain and Nerve Health

1. **Ginkgo Biloba**:

- **Properties**: Cognitive enhancer, antioxidant, improves blood flow to the brain.
- **Usage**: Ginkgo Biloba can be taken as a supplement or tea to improve memory, concentration, and overall brain function.

2. **Bacopa Monnieri**:
    - **Properties**: Neuroprotective, memory enhancer, reduces anxiety.
    - **Usage**: Bacopa is commonly used in Ayurvedic medicine to enhance cognitive function and reduce stress. It can be taken as a supplement or in powder form.

3. **Ashwagandha (Withania somnifera)**:
    - **Properties**: Adaptogen, neuroprotective, reduces stress and anxiety.
    - **Usage**: Ashwagandha can be taken as a capsule, tincture, or powder. It helps in reducing stress and supporting brain function.

4. **Gotu Kola (Centella asiatica)**:
    - **Properties**: Cognitive enhancer, anti-anxiety, improves circulation.
    - **Usage**: Gotu Kola is often used to enhance memory and cognitive function, and can be taken as a tea, tincture, or supplement.

5. **Lion's Mane Mushroom (Hericium erinaceus)**:
    - **Properties**: Neuroprotective, supports nerve regeneration, enhances cognitive function.
    - **Usage**: Lion's Mane can be taken as a supplement or added to teas and foods to support brain health and nerve regeneration.

Dietary Recommendations

1. **Antioxidant-Rich Foods**:
    - **Purpose**: Antioxidants help protect the brain from oxidative stress, which can lead to cognitive decline.
    - **Include**:
        - **Berries**: Blueberries, strawberries, and blackberries are rich in antioxidants like flavonoids.
        - **Dark Chocolate**: Contains flavonoids that improve brain function.
        - **Nuts and Seeds**: Almonds, walnuts, and flaxseeds are rich in vitamin E, an antioxidant that supports brain health.

2. **Healthy Fats**:
   - **Purpose**: Healthy fats are essential for brain structure and function.
   - **Include**:
     - **Omega-3 Fatty Acids**: Found in fatty fish (salmon, mackerel), flaxseeds, and walnuts. Omega-3s support brain function and reduce inflammation.
     - **Avocado**: Provides healthy monounsaturated fats that support brain health.

3. **Brain-Boosting Nutrients**:
   - **B-Vitamins**: Especially B6, B9 (folate), and B12 are crucial for brain function and nerve health. Include foods like leafy greens, eggs, and legumes.
   - **Choline**: Found in eggs, liver, and soybeans, choline is essential for memory and cognitive function.
   - **Magnesium**: Found in leafy greens, nuts, and seeds, magnesium supports nerve function and helps reduce stress.

4. **Hydration**:
   - **Importance**: Staying hydrated is vital for cognitive function. Drink plenty of water, herbal teas, and hydrating foods like cucumbers and melons.

5. **Blood Sugar Regulation**:
   - **Purpose**: Stable blood sugar levels are important for brain health and cognitive function.
   - **Include**: Whole grains, legumes, and low-glycemic fruits like berries and apples.

Exercise and Physical Activity

1. **Aerobic Exercise**:
   - **Benefits**: Increases blood flow to the brain, promotes the growth of new neurons, and improves overall cognitive function.
   - **Examples**: Brisk walking, running, swimming, and cycling. Aim for at least 150 minutes of moderate-intensity aerobic activity per week.

2. **Strength Training**:
   - **Benefits**: Improves brain function by increasing the release of brain-derived neurotrophic factor (BDNF), which supports neuron growth.

- **Examples**: Weight lifting, resistance band exercises, or bodyweight exercises like squats and push-ups.

3. **Mind-Body Exercises**:
   - **Yoga**: Enhances brain function by reducing stress and improving focus.
   - **Tai Chi**: Improves balance, coordination, and mental clarity while reducing stress.

4. **Mental Exercises**:
   - **Cognitive Training**: Engage in activities that challenge the brain, such as puzzles, memory games, and learning new skills or languages.

Lifestyle Changes

1. **Stress Management**:
   - **Meditation**: Regular practice can reduce stress, improve concentration, and enhance overall brain function.
   - **Deep Breathing**: Helps to reduce stress and anxiety, promoting a calm mind.
   - **Mindfulness**: Practicing mindfulness helps improve focus and mental clarity.

2. **Sleep Hygiene**:
   - **Importance**: Sleep is critical for memory consolidation and cognitive function. Aim for 7-9 hours of quality sleep per night.
   - **Tips**: Create a relaxing bedtime routine, avoid screens before bed, and keep your sleep environment dark and cool.

3. **Social Engagement**:
   - **Benefits**: Social interactions stimulate cognitive function and reduce the risk of cognitive decline.
   - **Activities**: Engage in regular social activities, join clubs or groups, and maintain close relationships with friends and family.

4. **Cognitive Stimulation**:
   - **Lifelong Learning**: Continue to challenge your brain by learning new skills, taking up new hobbies, or engaging in educational activities.
   - **Reading and Writing**: Regular reading and journaling can help maintain cognitive function and mental clarity.

Additional Therapies

1. **Acupuncture**:
   - **Benefits**: Can help reduce stress, improve focus, and support overall brain health by balancing energy in the body.

2. **Massage Therapy**:
   - **Usage**: Regular massage can help reduce stress and improve circulation, which is beneficial for brain function.

3. **Cold Showers or Cryotherapy**:
   - **Benefits**: Cold exposure can stimulate the release of norepinephrine, a neurotransmitter that supports focus and alertness.

4. **Brainwave Entrainment**:
   - **Usage**: Using sound or light pulses to synchronize brainwave frequencies can enhance cognitive function, relaxation, and focus.

Conclusion

Maintaining brain and nerve health is essential for a long, vibrant life. By integrating herbal remedies, proper nutrition, regular exercise, and lifestyle changes, you can support cognitive function, protect against neurodegenerative diseases, and promote overall neurological well-being. Regular practice of these protocols will help keep your brain sharp and your nerves healthy. Always consult with a healthcare provider before starting any new treatment plan, especially if you have pre-existing conditions or are taking other medications.

Gastroesophageal Reflux Disease (GERD) and Acid Reflux

Gastroesophageal Reflux Disease (GERD) and acid reflux occur when stomach acid flows back into the esophagus, causing irritation and discomfort. Managing GERD and acid reflux effectively requires a holistic approach, including dietary changes, herbal remedies, lifestyle adjustments, and stress management techniques to reduce symptoms and prevent long-term complications.

Key Herbs for GERD and Acid Reflux Management

1. **Licorice Root (Glycyrrhiza glabra)**:
   - **Properties**: Soothing, anti-inflammatory, protects the mucous membranes.
   - **Usage**: Deglycyrrhizinated licorice (DGL) can be taken as a chewable tablet or in powder form before meals to help soothe and protect the esophagus from stomach acid.

2. **Slippery Elm (Ulmus rubra)**:

- **Properties**: Demulcent, forms a protective barrier in the esophagus, anti-inflammatory.
- **Usage**: Slippery Elm can be taken as a powder mixed with water or as a tea to coat the lining of the esophagus and reduce irritation from acid reflux.

3. **Marshmallow Root (Althaea officinalis)**:
   - **Properties**: Demulcent, soothing, anti-inflammatory.
   - **Usage**: Marshmallow root tea or tincture can be taken before meals to soothe the digestive tract and reduce reflux symptoms.

4. **Chamomile (Matricaria chamomilla)**:
   - **Properties**: Anti-inflammatory, calming, digestive aid.
   - **Usage**: Chamomile tea can be consumed regularly to help reduce inflammation in the digestive tract and promote relaxation, which can reduce symptoms of GERD.

5. **Ginger (Zingiber officinale)**:
   - **Properties**: Digestive aid, anti-inflammatory, reduces nausea.
   - **Usage**: Ginger can be taken as a tea, in capsule form, or added to meals to help reduce acid reflux symptoms and improve digestion.

Dietary Recommendations

1. **Alkaline Foods**:
   - **Purpose**: Alkaline foods can help neutralize stomach acid and reduce symptoms.
   - **Include**:
     - **Leafy Greens**: Spinach, kale, and arugula are alkaline and help balance stomach acid.
     - **Cucumbers**: Hydrating and alkaline, cucumbers can soothe the digestive tract.
     - **Melons**: Cantaloupe and honeydew have high water content and are alkaline, which can help reduce acidity.

2. **Small, Frequent Meals**:
   - **Purpose**: Eating smaller meals more frequently can prevent the stomach from becoming too full and reduce the likelihood of acid reflux.

- **Tips**: Avoid overeating and aim for five to six small meals throughout the day.

3. **Avoid Trigger Foods**:
   - **Common Triggers**:
     - **Spicy Foods**: Can irritate the esophagus and worsen symptoms.
     - **Citrus Fruits**: High in acid, they can aggravate reflux.
     - **Tomato-Based Foods**: Tomatoes are acidic and can increase acid reflux.
     - **Fried and Fatty Foods**: Slow down digestion and increase the risk of reflux.
     - **Chocolate and Caffeine**: Can relax the lower esophageal sphincter, allowing acid to escape from the stomach into the esophagus.

4. **Hydration**:
   - **Importance**: Drink plenty of water throughout the day to help dilute stomach acid. Avoid drinking large amounts of water with meals, as this can exacerbate reflux.

5. **Mindful Eating**:
   - **Practice**: Eat slowly and chew your food thoroughly to promote better digestion and reduce the likelihood of acid reflux.

Exercise and Physical Activity

1. **Gentle Physical Activity**:
   - **Benefits**: Regular exercise can help maintain a healthy weight, which is crucial for managing GERD symptoms.
   - **Examples**: Walking, cycling, swimming, and yoga. Avoid high-impact exercises that can increase pressure on the abdomen and exacerbate reflux.

2. **Post-Meal Activity**:
   - **Walking**: Taking a gentle walk after meals can help stimulate digestion and prevent reflux. Avoid lying down immediately after eating.

Lifestyle Changes

1. **Elevate the Head of Your Bed**:
   - **Purpose**: Elevating the head of your bed by 6 to 8 inches can prevent stomach acid from flowing back into the esophagus while you sleep.

- **Tips**: Use a wedge pillow or place blocks under the legs of the bed at the head end.

2. **Weight Management**:
    - **Importance**: Maintaining a healthy weight can reduce pressure on the abdomen and lower the risk of acid reflux.

3. **Avoid Lying Down After Meals**:
    - **Guideline**: Wait at least 2-3 hours after eating before lying down to prevent stomach acid from flowing back into the esophagus.

4. **Quit Smoking**:
    - **Impact**: Smoking weakens the lower esophageal sphincter, making acid reflux more likely. Quitting smoking can significantly improve GERD symptoms.

5. **Stress Management**:
    - **Meditation and Relaxation**: Regular practice of meditation and deep breathing exercises can reduce stress, which is a known trigger for acid reflux.
    - **Journaling**: Keeping a food and symptom diary can help identify triggers and improve management of GERD.

Additional Therapies

1. **Acupuncture**:
    - **Benefits**: Can help reduce symptoms of GERD by balancing energy flow and improving digestive function.

2. **Probiotics**:
    - **Usage**: Taking a probiotic supplement can help balance gut bacteria, improving digestion and potentially reducing acid reflux.

3. **Digestive Enzymes**:
    - **Usage**: Supplementing with digestive enzymes can aid in breaking down food more efficiently, reducing the likelihood of acid reflux.

4. **Apple Cider Vinegar**:
    - **Usage**: A small amount of diluted apple cider vinegar before meals may help balance stomach acidity. However, this should be approached cautiously and discussed with a healthcare provider, as it may not be suitable for everyone.

Conclusion

Managing GERD and acid reflux involves a comprehensive approach that includes herbal remedies, dietary adjustments, regular exercise, and key lifestyle changes. By addressing the underlying causes of acid reflux and adopting these natural strategies, you can significantly reduce symptoms, improve digestion, and enhance your quality of life. Always consult with a healthcare provider before starting any new treatment plan, especially if you have a chronic condition or are taking other medications.

Prostate Health

Prostate health is crucial for men, particularly as they age, to prevent conditions such as benign prostatic hyperplasia (BPH), prostatitis, and prostate cancer. This protocol offers a holistic approach that includes herbal remedies, dietary strategies, lifestyle changes, and specific exercises to support and maintain a healthy prostate.

Key Herbs for Prostate Health

1. **Saw Palmetto (Serenoa repens)**:
    - **Properties**: Anti-inflammatory, supports healthy hormone levels, helps reduce symptoms of BPH.
    - **Usage**: Saw Palmetto is commonly taken as a supplement or tincture to promote prostate health and reduce urinary symptoms associated with an enlarged prostate.

2. **Stinging Nettle Root (Urtica dioica)**:
    - **Properties**: Anti-inflammatory, supports urinary tract health, helps manage symptoms of BPH.
    - **Usage**: Stinging Nettle Root can be taken as a tea, tincture, or supplement to reduce urinary symptoms and support overall prostate health.

3. **Pygeum (Pygeum africanum)**:
    - **Properties**: Anti-inflammatory, improves urinary symptoms, supports prostate health.
    - **Usage**: Pygeum is typically taken as a supplement and is known for its effectiveness in reducing symptoms of BPH and improving urinary flow.

4. **Pumpkin Seed Oil (Cucurbita pepo)**:
    - **Properties**: Rich in essential fatty acids and antioxidants, supports prostate function.

- **Usage**: Pumpkin seed oil can be consumed directly or in capsule form to support prostate health and reduce symptoms of BPH.

5. **Rye Grass Pollen (Secale cereale)**:
    - **Properties**: Supports urinary function, reduces inflammation, helps with symptoms of BPH.
    - **Usage**: Rye Grass Pollen extract is used as a supplement to help improve urinary flow and reduce prostate-related symptoms.

Dietary Recommendations

1. **Zinc-Rich Foods**:
    - **Importance**: Zinc is essential for prostate health and plays a role in maintaining normal hormone levels.
    - **Include**: Shellfish (especially oysters), pumpkin seeds, spinach, and nuts.

2. **Cruciferous Vegetables**:
    - **Purpose**: Cruciferous vegetables contain compounds that may reduce the risk of prostate cancer and promote overall prostate health.
    - **Include**: Broccoli, Brussels sprouts, kale, and cauliflower.

3. **Lycopene-Rich Foods**:
    - **Importance**: Lycopene is an antioxidant that supports prostate health and may reduce the risk of prostate cancer.
    - **Include**: Tomatoes (especially cooked or processed, like tomato sauce), watermelon, and pink grapefruit.

4. **Healthy Fats**:
    - **Focus on**: Omega-3 fatty acids, which help reduce inflammation and support overall prostate health.
    - **Include**: Fatty fish (salmon, mackerel), flaxseeds, and walnuts.

5. **Green Tea**:
    - **Properties**: Rich in antioxidants, green tea supports prostate health and may reduce the risk of prostate cancer.
    - **Usage**: Drink 1-2 cups of green tea daily to benefit from its protective effects.

6. **Limit Red Meat and Dairy**:

- **Reason**: High consumption of red meat and dairy products has been linked to an increased risk of prostate issues.
- **Recommendation**: Limit intake and focus on plant-based sources of protein and calcium.

Exercise and Physical Activity

1. **Regular Aerobic Exercise**:
   - **Benefits**: Helps maintain a healthy weight, reduce inflammation, and improve overall prostate health.
   - **Examples**: Brisk walking, jogging, swimming, and cycling. Aim for at least 150 minutes of moderate-intensity exercise per week.

2. **Pelvic Floor Exercises (Kegels)**:
   - **Purpose**: Strengthen the pelvic floor muscles, which can improve urinary control and support prostate health.
   - **Practice**: Contract the muscles you would use to stop the flow of urine, hold for a few seconds, and then release. Repeat several times a day.

3. **Resistance Training**:
   - **Benefits**: Helps maintain muscle mass, improve metabolism, and support overall health.
   - **Examples**: Weight lifting, resistance bands, or bodyweight exercises like squats and lunges.

Lifestyle Changes

1. **Regular Medical Check-Ups**:
   - **Importance**: Regular screenings, including prostate-specific antigen (PSA) tests, are crucial for early detection and management of prostate issues.
   - **Recommendation**: Men over the age of 50 (or younger if at higher risk) should have regular prostate screenings.

2. **Stress Management**:
   - **Meditation and Mindfulness**: Reducing stress can lower inflammation and support overall health. Practices like meditation, deep breathing, and mindfulness can help manage stress levels.
   - **Relaxation Techniques**: Engage in activities that promote relaxation, such as yoga, tai chi, or spending time in nature.

3. **Hydration**:
   - **Importance**: Adequate hydration supports urinary tract health and can help flush out toxins that could affect the prostate.
   - **Guideline**: Drink plenty of water throughout the day, but reduce intake in the evening to minimize nighttime urination.
4. **Healthy Weight Maintenance**:
   - **Reason**: Excess weight can increase the risk of prostate problems, including BPH and prostate cancer.
   - **Approach**: Maintain a balanced diet and regular exercise routine to keep weight within a healthy range.

Additional Therapies

1. **Acupuncture**:
   - **Benefits**: May help reduce symptoms of prostatitis and improve overall prostate health by balancing energy flow and reducing inflammation.
2. **Massage Therapy**:
   - **Usage**: Regular prostate massage, when performed by a trained professional, can help relieve symptoms of prostatitis and support prostate health.
3. **Herbal Supplements**:
   - **Combination Formulas**: Some supplements combine several prostate-supporting herbs (like saw palmetto, pygeum, and stinging nettle) for enhanced effects.
4. **Heat Therapy**:
   - **Usage**: Applying heat to the lower abdomen can help relieve discomfort associated with prostate issues, such as prostatitis.

Conclusion

Supporting prostate health involves a comprehensive approach that includes the use of specific herbs, dietary modifications, regular exercise, and lifestyle adjustments. These strategies can help prevent and manage common prostate issues, promote overall urinary health, and reduce the risk of prostate-related diseases. Always consult with a healthcare provider before starting any new treatment plan, especially if you have existing health conditions or are taking other medications.

Lung Health and Chronic Obstructive Pulmonary Disease (COPD)

Maintaining lung health is crucial for overall well-being, particularly for those at risk of or suffering from Chronic Obstructive Pulmonary Disease (COPD). This protocol focuses on herbal remedies, dietary strategies, breathing exercises, and lifestyle changes to support lung function, reduce inflammation, and manage symptoms associated with COPD.

Key Herbs for Lung Health and COPD

1. **Mullein (Verbascum thapsus)**:
   - **Properties**: Expectorant, anti-inflammatory, soothes the respiratory tract.
   - **Usage**: Mullein can be taken as a tea or tincture to help clear mucus from the lungs and reduce inflammation.

2. **Lobelia (Lobelia inflata)**:
   - **Properties**: Bronchodilator, antispasmodic, helps open airways.
   - **Usage**: Lobelia tincture can be used in small doses to help relieve bronchial spasms and improve breathing in those with COPD.

3. **Elecampane (Inula helenium)**:
   - **Properties**: Expectorant, antimicrobial, supports lung health.
   - **Usage**: Elecampane root can be taken as a tea or tincture to help clear mucus from the lungs and support respiratory health.

4. **Thyme (Thymus vulgaris)**:
   - **Properties**: Antimicrobial, expectorant, supports immune function.
   - **Usage**: Thyme can be used in teas or as an essential oil (inhaled) to help clear mucus and fight respiratory infections.

5. **Peppermint (Mentha piperita)**:
   - **Properties**: Decongestant, antispasmodic, soothes the respiratory tract.
   - **Usage**: Peppermint tea or essential oil (inhaled) can help open airways, reduce congestion, and improve breathing.

6. **Ginger (Zingiber officinale)**:
   - **Properties**: Anti-inflammatory, antioxidant, helps reduce bronchial inflammation.

- **Usage**: Ginger tea or capsules can be used to reduce inflammation in the lungs and support overall respiratory health.

Dietary Recommendations

1. **Anti-Inflammatory Foods**:
   - **Importance**: Reducing inflammation is crucial for managing COPD and improving lung function.
   - **Include**:
     - **Fatty Fish**: Salmon, mackerel, and sardines are rich in omega-3 fatty acids, which help reduce inflammation.
     - **Berries**: Blueberries, strawberries, and raspberries are high in antioxidants that support lung health.
     - **Leafy Greens**: Spinach, kale, and arugula are rich in vitamins and minerals that support respiratory health.

2. **Foods Rich in Vitamin C**:
   - **Purpose**: Vitamin C is essential for lung health and supports immune function.
   - **Include**: Oranges, bell peppers, strawberries, and broccoli.

3. **Hydration**:
   - **Importance**: Staying well-hydrated helps thin mucus, making it easier to clear from the lungs.
   - **Guideline**: Drink plenty of water throughout the day, and consider herbal teas that support respiratory health.

4. **Limit Dairy and Processed Foods**:
   - **Reason**: Dairy and processed foods can increase mucus production and exacerbate COPD symptoms.
   - **Recommendation**: Reduce or eliminate these foods from your diet to improve lung function.

5. **Magnesium-Rich Foods**:
   - **Importance**: Magnesium helps relax bronchial muscles, improving lung function.
   - **Include**: Nuts, seeds, spinach, and black beans.

6. **Garlic and Onions**:

- **Properties**: Both are natural anti-inflammatories and can help reduce respiratory inflammation.
- **Usage**: Incorporate raw or cooked garlic and onions into meals to support lung health.

Breathing Exercises

1. **Pursed-Lip Breathing**:
    - **Purpose**: Helps reduce shortness of breath by slowing down breathing and improving oxygen exchange.
    - **Practice**:
        - Inhale slowly through your nose for two counts.
        - Purse your lips as if you are going to whistle.
        - Exhale slowly and gently through your pursed lips for four counts.
        - Repeat several times, especially during activities that cause shortness of breath.

2. **Diaphragmatic Breathing (Belly Breathing)**:
    - **Purpose**: Strengthens the diaphragm and promotes deeper, more efficient breathing.
    - **Practice**:
        - Sit or lie down in a comfortable position.
        - Place one hand on your chest and the other on your abdomen.
        - Breathe in slowly through your nose, allowing your abdomen to rise while keeping your chest still.
        - Exhale slowly through pursed lips, letting your abdomen fall.
        - Practice this for 5-10 minutes daily.

3. **Controlled Coughing**:
    - **Purpose**: Helps clear mucus from the lungs, which is essential for COPD management.
    - **Practice**:
        - Sit in a comfortable chair and lean slightly forward.
        - Inhale deeply through your nose.

- Cough twice, keeping your mouth slightly open. The first cough loosens mucus, and the second helps to expel it.
- Rest and repeat as needed.

Lifestyle Changes

1. **Avoid Smoking and Secondhand Smoke**:
   - **Importance**: Smoking is the leading cause of COPD. Quitting smoking and avoiding secondhand smoke are crucial for lung health.
   - **Resources**: Seek support through cessation programs, counseling, and nicotine replacement therapies.

2. **Air Quality**:
   - **Guidelines**:
     - Use air purifiers in your home to reduce exposure to pollutants and allergens.
     - Monitor local air quality reports and avoid outdoor activities on days when pollution levels are high.
     - Ventilate your living spaces to reduce indoor pollutants.

3. **Regular Physical Activity**:
   - **Benefits**: Exercise improves overall health, strengthens respiratory muscles, and enhances lung capacity.
   - **Examples**: Walking, swimming, or cycling. Incorporate low-impact exercises that do not strain your lungs.

4. **Healthy Weight Maintenance**:
   - **Reason**: Excess weight can make breathing more difficult and exacerbate COPD symptoms.
   - **Approach**: Maintain a balanced diet and regular exercise routine to achieve or maintain a healthy weight.

5. **Pulmonary Rehabilitation**:
   - **Purpose**: A comprehensive program that includes exercise, education, and support to improve lung function and quality of life for COPD patients.
   - **Recommendation**: Consider enrolling in a pulmonary rehabilitation program under the guidance of healthcare professionals.

Additional Therapies

1. **Steam Inhalation**:
    - **Usage**: Inhaling steam can help loosen mucus and make it easier to expel from the lungs.
    - **Practice**: Add a few drops of eucalyptus or peppermint essential oil to a bowl of hot water, lean over the bowl with a towel over your head, and inhale the steam for 5-10 minutes.
2. **Chest Percussion**:
    - **Technique**: This involves tapping on the chest and back to help loosen mucus in the lungs, making it easier to cough up.
    - **Guidance**: Chest percussion is often performed by a respiratory therapist, but it can be taught to family members or caregivers.
3. **Essential Oils**:
    - **Options**: Eucalyptus, peppermint, and tea tree oils can be used in diffusers or applied topically (diluted with a carrier oil) to support respiratory health.
4. **Humidifiers**:
    - **Purpose**: Keeping the air moist can help ease breathing and prevent the airways from drying out.
    - **Usage**: Use a humidifier in your home, especially during dry weather or winter months, to maintain optimal humidity levels.

Conclusion

Managing lung health and COPD requires a multi-faceted approach that includes herbal remedies, dietary strategies, regular breathing exercises, and key lifestyle changes. By adopting these holistic strategies, you can improve lung function, reduce symptoms, and enhance your overall quality of life. Always consult with a healthcare provider before starting any new treatment plan, especially if you have a chronic condition or are taking other medications.

Parkinson's Disease

Parkinson's Disease is a progressive neurological disorder characterized by tremors, rigidity, bradykinesia (slowness of movement), and postural instability. Managing Parkinson's Disease holistically involves integrating herbal remedies, dietary adjustments, physical activity, and lifestyle changes to support overall health, manage symptoms, and improve quality of life.

Key Herbs for Parkinson's Disease

1. **Turmeric (Curcuma longa)**:
   - **Properties**: Anti-inflammatory, antioxidant, supports brain health.
   - **Usage**: Turmeric can be taken as a spice in foods, as a tea, or in supplement form (curcumin) to help reduce inflammation and oxidative stress associated with Parkinson's Disease.

2. **Gingko Biloba (Gingko biloba)**:
   - **Properties**: Antioxidant, improves cognitive function, supports circulation.
   - **Usage**: Gingko Biloba extract can be taken as a supplement to help improve cognitive function and reduce symptoms of Parkinson's Disease.

3. **Ashwagandha (Withania somnifera)**:
   - **Properties**: Adaptogen, helps manage stress, supports neurological health.
   - **Usage**: Ashwagandha can be taken as a powder or in supplement form to help manage stress and support overall brain health.

4. **Rhodiola (Rhodiola rosea)**:
   - **Properties**: Adaptogen, enhances mental clarity, reduces fatigue.
   - **Usage**: Rhodiola can be taken as a supplement to improve mental clarity and reduce fatigue associated with Parkinson's Disease.

5. **Green Tea (Camellia sinensis)**:
   - **Properties**: Antioxidant, supports brain health, reduces oxidative stress.
   - **Usage**: Drinking green tea regularly can help reduce oxidative stress and support overall brain health.

6. **Gotu Kola (Centella asiatica)**:
   - **Properties**: Supports cognitive function, improves circulation.
   - **Usage**: Gotu Kola can be taken as a tea or in supplement form to support cognitive function and improve circulation.

Dietary Recommendations

1. **Antioxidant-Rich Foods**:
   - **Purpose**: Antioxidants help combat oxidative stress, which is involved in the progression of Parkinson's Disease.
   - **Include**:
     - **Berries**: Blueberries, strawberries, and raspberries.

- **Leafy Greens**: Spinach, kale, and Swiss chard.
- **Nuts and Seeds**: Walnuts, almonds, and chia seeds.

2. **Omega-3 Fatty Acids**:
   - **Importance**: Omega-3s support brain health and have anti-inflammatory properties.
   - **Include**: Fatty fish (salmon, mackerel), flaxseeds, chia seeds, and walnuts.

3. **Fiber-Rich Foods**:
   - **Purpose**: Fiber helps manage digestive issues, which can be a concern in Parkinson's Disease.
   - **Include**: Whole grains, fruits, vegetables, legumes, and nuts.

4. **Hydration**:
   - **Importance**: Adequate hydration is essential for maintaining overall health and managing symptoms.
   - **Guideline**: Drink plenty of water throughout the day, and consider herbal teas that support brain health.

5. **Limit Processed Foods and Sugars**:
   - **Reason**: Processed foods and high sugar intake can contribute to inflammation and exacerbate symptoms.
   - **Recommendation**: Focus on whole, unprocessed foods and reduce intake of sugary snacks and beverages.

6. **Vitamin D and B Vitamins**:
   - **Importance**: Vitamin D supports brain health and immune function, while B vitamins are crucial for energy and cognitive function.
   - **Include**:
     - **Vitamin D**: Sun exposure, fortified foods, and supplements.
     - **B Vitamins**: Whole grains, legumes, meat, eggs, and dairy.

Physical Activity and Exercise

1. **Regular Aerobic Exercise**:
   - **Benefits**: Improves cardiovascular health, supports mobility, and enhances overall well-being.

- **Examples**: Walking, swimming, cycling, and dancing. Aim for at least 150 minutes of moderate-intensity exercise per week.

2. **Strength Training**:
    - **Purpose**: Helps maintain muscle strength and balance, which is important for managing Parkinson's Disease.
    - **Examples**: Resistance exercises, weight lifting, or bodyweight exercises like squats and lunges.

3. **Flexibility and Stretching**:
    - **Benefits**: Improves range of motion and reduces stiffness.
    - **Examples**: Yoga or Pilates can help maintain flexibility and support overall physical function.

4. **Balance and Coordination Exercises**:
    - **Purpose**: Helps prevent falls and improves stability.
    - **Examples**: Tai Chi, balance exercises, and stability training.

5. **Speech and Swallowing Exercises**:
    - **Importance**: As Parkinson's Disease progresses, speech and swallowing can become affected.
    - **Recommendation**: Work with a speech therapist for targeted exercises to maintain communication skills and manage swallowing difficulties.

Lifestyle Changes

1. **Stress Management**:
    - **Importance**: Managing stress can help improve symptoms and quality of life.
    - **Techniques**: Practice relaxation techniques such as meditation, deep breathing, and mindfulness.

2. **Adequate Sleep**:
    - **Importance**: Quality sleep is essential for overall health and symptom management.
    - **Guideline**: Establish a regular sleep routine and create a restful sleep environment.

3. **Support Networks**:

- **Purpose**: Emotional and social support can significantly impact quality of life.
- **Recommendation**: Join support groups for individuals with Parkinson's Disease and engage with family and friends for emotional support.

4. **Cognitive Stimulation**:
    - **Importance**: Engaging in activities that stimulate the brain can help maintain cognitive function.
    - **Examples**: Puzzles, reading, learning new skills, and engaging in creative hobbies.

5. **Avoid Toxins**:
    - **Reason**: Exposure to environmental toxins may exacerbate Parkinson's Disease symptoms.
    - **Guideline**: Minimize exposure to pollutants, chemicals, and pesticides.

Additional Therapies

1. **Acupuncture**:
    - **Benefits**: May help reduce symptoms such as tremors, rigidity, and pain associated with Parkinson's Disease.

2. **Massage Therapy**:
    - **Usage**: Regular massage can help alleviate muscle stiffness and improve circulation.

3. **Music Therapy**:
    - **Purpose**: Engaging with music can improve mood, motor function, and overall well-being.
    - **Practice**: Participate in music therapy sessions or enjoy music as part of daily life.

4. **Art Therapy**:
    - **Benefits**: Art therapy can provide emotional expression and cognitive stimulation.

Conclusion

Managing Parkinson's Disease holistically involves a comprehensive approach that includes herbal remedies, dietary adjustments, regular exercise, and lifestyle changes. By adopting these strategies, you can support brain health, manage symptoms, and improve your overall quality of life. Always consult with a healthcare provider before starting any new treatment plan, especially if you have a chronic condition or are taking other medications.

Type-2 Diabetes

Type-2 Diabetes is a chronic condition characterized by high blood sugar levels due to insulin resistance or inadequate insulin production. Managing Type-2 Diabetes holistically involves incorporating dietary changes, herbal remedies, exercise, and lifestyle adjustments to help control blood sugar levels and support overall health.

Key Herbs for Type-2 Diabetes

1. **Cinnamon (Cinnamomum verum)**:
   - **Properties**: Helps improve insulin sensitivity, lowers blood sugar levels.
   - **Usage**: Cinnamon can be added to foods and beverages or taken as a supplement to help manage blood sugar levels.

2. **Bitter Melon (Momordica charantia)**:
   - **Properties**: Contains compounds that mimic insulin and may lower blood sugar levels.
   - **Usage**: Bitter melon can be consumed as a vegetable, juice, or supplement to help manage diabetes.

3. **Fenugreek (Trigonella foenum-graecum)**:
   - **Properties**: Contains soluble fiber, which helps control blood sugar levels.
   - **Usage**: Fenugreek seeds can be used in cooking or taken as a supplement to help manage Type-2 Diabetes.

4. **Berberine (Berberis spp.)**:
   - **Properties**: Supports insulin sensitivity and helps regulate blood sugar levels.
   - **Usage**: Berberine is typically taken as a supplement to help manage Type-2 Diabetes.

5. **Ginseng (Panax ginseng)**:
   - **Properties**: May help improve insulin sensitivity and lower blood sugar levels.
   - **Usage**: Ginseng can be taken as a supplement or in tea form to support diabetes management.

6. **Turmeric (Curcuma longa)**:
    - **Properties**: Anti-inflammatory and may help improve insulin sensitivity.
    - **Usage**: Turmeric can be added to foods, taken as a supplement, or consumed as a tea.

Dietary Recommendations

1. **Low-Glycemic Index Foods**:
    - **Purpose**: Helps manage blood sugar levels by preventing rapid spikes.
    - **Include**:
        - **Non-Starchy Vegetables**: Leafy greens, broccoli, and peppers.
        - **Whole Grains**: Quinoa, barley, and brown rice.
        - **Legumes**: Beans, lentils, and chickpeas.
2. **High-Fiber Foods**:
    - **Importance**: Fiber helps regulate blood sugar levels and supports digestive health.
    - **Include**: Fruits, vegetables, whole grains, nuts, and seeds.
3. **Lean Proteins**:
    - **Purpose**: Supports muscle mass and helps with blood sugar control.
    - **Include**: Skinless poultry, fish, tofu, legumes, and low-fat dairy products.
4. **Healthy Fats**:
    - **Importance**: Provides energy and supports heart health.
    - **Include**: Avocado, nuts, seeds, and olive oil.
5. **Limit Added Sugars and Refined Carbohydrates**:
    - **Reason**: These can cause rapid spikes in blood sugar levels.
    - **Recommendation**: Avoid sugary snacks, beverages, and refined grains.
6. **Stay Hydrated**:
    - **Importance**: Proper hydration is essential for overall health and blood sugar management.
    - **Guideline**: Drink plenty of water throughout the day. Herbal teas like green tea can also be beneficial.

7. **Control Portion Sizes**:
   - **Purpose**: Helps prevent overeating and manage blood sugar levels.
   - **Strategy**: Use smaller plates, pay attention to hunger cues, and avoid eating large meals.

Physical Activity and Exercise

1. **Regular Aerobic Exercise**:
   - **Benefits**: Helps improve insulin sensitivity and supports weight management.
   - **Examples**: Walking, cycling, swimming, or jogging. Aim for at least 150 minutes of moderate-intensity exercise per week.

2. **Strength Training**:
   - **Purpose**: Builds muscle mass, which can improve blood sugar control.
   - **Examples**: Weight lifting, resistance band exercises, or bodyweight exercises like squats and lunges.

3. **Flexibility and Stretching**:
   - **Benefits**: Enhances mobility and reduces muscle stiffness.
   - **Examples**: Yoga, stretching exercises, and Pilates.

4. **Balance and Coordination Exercises**:
   - **Purpose**: Helps prevent falls and improves overall stability.
   - **Examples**: Balance exercises, Tai Chi, and stability training.

5. **Regular Physical Activity**:
   - **Importance**: Consistency in physical activity helps maintain blood sugar levels and overall health.
   - **Guideline**: Incorporate exercise into daily routines, such as walking after meals or using stairs instead of elevators.

Lifestyle Changes

1. **Stress Management**:
   - **Importance**: Chronic stress can affect blood sugar levels and overall health.
   - **Techniques**: Practice relaxation techniques like deep breathing, meditation, and mindfulness.

2. **Regular Sleep**:
    - **Importance**: Quality sleep supports overall health and blood sugar control.
    - **Guideline**: Aim for 7-9 hours of sleep per night and establish a regular sleep routine.
3. **Monitoring Blood Sugar Levels**:
    - **Purpose**: Regular monitoring helps manage diabetes and make necessary adjustments.
    - **Recommendation**: Use a glucose meter as recommended by your healthcare provider to track blood sugar levels.
4. **Support Networks**:
    - **Purpose**: Emotional and social support can impact diabetes management.
    - **Recommendation**: Join diabetes support groups and engage with family and friends for encouragement and support.
5. **Avoid Smoking and Limit Alcohol**:
    - **Reason**: Smoking and excessive alcohol consumption can negatively impact blood sugar levels and overall health.
    - **Guideline**: Avoid smoking and limit alcohol intake to moderate levels.

Additional Therapies

1. **Acupuncture**:
    - **Benefits**: May help improve insulin sensitivity and regulate blood sugar levels.
2. **Yoga and Mindfulness**:
    - **Usage**: Yoga and mindfulness practices can help reduce stress and improve overall well-being.
3. **Cinnamon Supplements**:
    - **Purpose**: Specific supplements may provide higher doses of cinnamon to support blood sugar management.
4. **Biofeedback**:
    - **Benefits**: Can help individuals learn to manage stress and physiological responses that affect blood sugar levels.

Conclusion

Managing Type-2 Diabetes holistically involves a comprehensive approach that includes dietary changes, herbal remedies, regular exercise, and lifestyle adjustments. By adopting these strategies, you can support blood sugar control, improve overall health, and enhance your quality of life. Always consult with a healthcare provider before starting any new treatment plan or making significant changes to your current regimen.

Leaky Gut, Gastritis, and Irritable Bowel Syndrome (IBS)

Leaky Gut Syndrome, Gastritis, and Irritable Bowel Syndrome (IBS) are common digestive disorders that can significantly impact quality of life. Managing these conditions holistically involves using herbal remedies, dietary adjustments, lifestyle changes, and supportive therapies to address underlying causes, reduce symptoms, and promote gut health.

Leaky Gut Syndrome

Leaky Gut Syndrome is a condition where the intestinal lining becomes more permeable, allowing toxins and undigested food particles to enter the bloodstream, leading to inflammation and immune responses.

Key Herbs for Leaky Gut Syndrome:

1. **Slippery Elm (Ulmus rubra)**:
   - **Properties**: Soothes and protects the mucous membranes of the digestive tract.
   - **Usage**: Taken as a tea or in powder form to help soothe and heal the gut lining.

2. **Marshmallow Root (Althaea officinalis)**:
   - **Properties**: Anti-inflammatory, mucilaginous, helps soothe the digestive tract.
   - **Usage**: Consumed as a tea or supplement to reduce inflammation and protect the gut lining.

3. **Licorice Root (Glycyrrhiza glabra)**:
   - **Properties**: Anti-inflammatory, supports mucosal health, helps with gut healing.
   - **Usage**: Used as a tea or in supplement form to support gut health and reduce inflammation.

4. **Aloe Vera (Aloe barbadensis)**:
   - **Properties**: Soothes the digestive tract, supports healing.

- **Usage**: Consumed as aloe vera juice to help soothe and heal the gut lining.
5. **Bone Broth**:
    - **Properties**: Contains amino acids and nutrients that support gut health and repair.
    - **Usage**: Consumed regularly as a nutrient-rich broth to support gut healing.

Dietary Recommendations for Leaky Gut Syndrome:
1. **Anti-Inflammatory Foods**:
    - **Purpose**: Reduce inflammation and support gut healing.
    - **Include**:
        - **Leafy Greens**: Spinach, kale, and Swiss chard.
        - **Fatty Fish**: Salmon, mackerel, and sardines.
        - **Turmeric and Ginger**: Anti-inflammatory spices.
2. **Gut-Healing Foods**:
    - **Importance**: Support the repair of the gut lining.
    - **Include**: Bone broth, fermented foods (kimchi, sauerkraut), and prebiotic foods (onions, garlic, bananas).
3. **Avoid Gluten and Dairy**:
    - **Reason**: Gluten and dairy can exacerbate symptoms and inflammation.
    - **Recommendation**: Opt for gluten-free grains and dairy-free alternatives.
4. **Low FODMAP Diet**:
    - **Purpose**: Reduces symptoms by eliminating fermentable carbohydrates that can cause digestive distress.
    - **Include**:
        - **Low FODMAP Foods**: Carrots, cucumbers, and zucchini.
        - **Avoid**: High FODMAP foods like onions, garlic, and apples.

Lifestyle Changes:
1. **Stress Management**:
    - **Importance**: Stress can worsen gut symptoms and inflammation.

- **Techniques**: Practice relaxation techniques like deep breathing, meditation, and yoga.

2. **Adequate Sleep**:
    - **Purpose**: Supports overall health and gut healing.
    - **Guideline**: Aim for 7-9 hours of quality sleep each night.

3. **Regular Exercise**:
    - **Benefits**: Enhances digestion and reduces stress.
    - **Examples**: Moderate exercise like walking, cycling, or swimming.

Gastritis

Gastritis is an inflammation of the stomach lining that can cause pain, nausea, and digestive discomfort.

Key Herbs for Gastritis:

1. **Chamomile (Matricaria chamomilla)**:
    - **Properties**: Anti-inflammatory, soothing to the stomach lining.
    - **Usage**: Consumed as tea to reduce inflammation and soothe the stomach.

2. **Peppermint (Mentha piperita)**:
    - **Properties**: Helps relieve nausea and indigestion.
    - **Usage**: Consumed as tea or in supplement form to help soothe digestive discomfort.

3. **Ginger (Zingiber officinale)**:
    - **Properties**: Anti-inflammatory, helps with nausea and digestive upset.
    - **Usage**: Consumed as tea, in cooking, or as a supplement.

4. **Marshmallow Root (Althaea officinalis)**:
    - **Properties**: Soothes and protects the stomach lining.
    - **Usage**: Taken as tea or supplement to reduce inflammation and protect the stomach lining.

Dietary Recommendations for Gastritis:

1. **Anti-Inflammatory Diet**:
    - **Purpose**: Reduces inflammation and supports healing.

- Include:
    - **Non-Spicy Foods**: Avoid spicy, acidic, or fried foods that can irritate the stomach lining.
    - **Gentle Foods**: Oatmeal, bananas, and cooked vegetables.
2. **Probiotics**:
    - **Importance**: Supports a healthy gut microbiome.
    - **Include**: Yogurt, kefir, and fermented vegetables.
3. **Avoid Alcohol and Caffeine**:
    - **Reason**: Both can irritate the stomach lining.
    - **Recommendation**: Limit or avoid alcohol and caffeine-containing beverages.
4. **Small, Frequent Meals**:
    - **Purpose**: Reduces stomach irritation and discomfort.
    - **Guideline**: Eat smaller meals more frequently throughout the day.

Lifestyle Changes:

1. **Stress Management**:
    - **Importance**: Stress can exacerbate gastritis symptoms.
    - **Techniques**: Practice relaxation techniques and manage stress effectively.
2. **Avoid Smoking**:
    - **Reason**: Smoking can aggravate gastritis and slow healing.
    - **Guideline**: Avoid smoking and exposure to tobacco smoke.

Irritable Bowel Syndrome (IBS)

IBS is a functional gastrointestinal disorder characterized by symptoms such as abdominal pain, bloating, and changes in bowel habits.

Key Herbs for IBS:

1. **Peppermint (Mentha piperita)**:
    - **Properties**: Relieves abdominal pain and bloating.
    - **Usage**: Consumed as tea or in enteric-coated capsules to help relieve IBS symptoms.
2. **Ginger (Zingiber officinale)**:

- **Properties**: Reduces nausea and digestive discomfort.
- **Usage**: Taken as tea or in supplement form to support digestion.

3. **Fennel Seeds (Foeniculum vulgare)**:
   - **Properties**: Helps reduce bloating and gas.
   - **Usage**: Chew fennel seeds or drink fennel tea to relieve IBS symptoms.

4. **Turmeric (Curcuma longa)**:
   - **Properties**: Anti-inflammatory, supports digestive health.
   - **Usage**: Can be added to foods or taken as a supplement.

5. **Slippery Elm (Ulmus rubra)**:
   - **Properties**: Soothes the digestive tract and supports gut health.
   - **Usage**: Consumed as a tea or powder to help manage IBS symptoms.

Dietary Recommendations for IBS:

1. **Low FODMAP Diet**:
   - **Purpose**: Reduces symptoms by eliminating fermentable carbohydrates.
   - **Include**:
     - **Low FODMAP Foods**: Carrots, rice, and spinach.
     - **Avoid**: High FODMAP foods like onions, garlic, and apples.

2. **Fiber Intake**:
   - **Importance**: Helps with bowel regularity.
   - **Include**: Soluble fiber sources like oats, psyllium husk, and chia seeds.

3. **Avoid Trigger Foods**:
   - **Reason**: Certain foods can exacerbate IBS symptoms.
   - **Recommendation**: Identify and avoid individual trigger foods, which may include fatty foods, dairy, or artificial sweeteners.

4. **Stay Hydrated**:
   - **Purpose**: Proper hydration supports digestive health.
   - **Guideline**: Drink plenty of water throughout the day and avoid excessive caffeine.

Lifestyle Changes:

1. **Regular Exercise**:
   - **Benefits**: Helps improve digestion and reduce stress.
   - **Examples**: Moderate exercise like walking, swimming, or cycling.
2. **Stress Management**:
   - **Importance**: Stress can trigger or worsen IBS symptoms.
   - **Techniques**: Practice relaxation techniques such as deep breathing, meditation, and mindfulness.
3. **Eating Mindfully**:
   - **Purpose**: Reduces digestive discomfort and supports better digestion.
   - **Guideline**: Eat slowly, chew food thoroughly, and avoid overeating.
4. **Keep a Food Diary**:
   - **Importance**: Helps identify trigger foods and manage symptoms.
   - **Practice**: Track foods, symptoms, and stress levels to identify patterns and make dietary adjustments.

Additional Therapies

1. **Acupuncture**:
   - **Benefits**: May help alleviate digestive discomfort and manage symptoms of IBS and gastritis.
2. **Probiotics**:
   - **Usage**: Can support gut health and balance the microbiome, potentially benefiting IBS and leaky gut.
3. **Biofeedback**:
   - **Purpose**: Helps manage stress and physiological responses that affect digestive health.
4. **Digestive Enzymes**:
   - **Benefits**: May aid in digestion and reduce symptoms of IBS.

Conclusion

Managing Leaky Gut Syndrome, Gastritis, and Irritable Bowel Syndrome (IBS) holistically involves a multi-faceted approach that includes herbal remedies, dietary changes, lifestyle adjustments, and supportive therapies. By incorporating these strategies, you can address underlying causes, alleviate symptoms, and promote overall digestive health. Always consult with a healthcare provider before starting any new treatment plan or making significant changes to your current regimen.

Lupus

Lupus is a chronic autoimmune disease where the immune system attacks healthy tissues, leading to inflammation and damage in various parts of the body, including the skin, joints, kidneys, and heart. Managing lupus holistically involves a combination of dietary adjustments, herbal remedies, lifestyle changes, and supportive therapies to help reduce symptoms, manage inflammation, and support overall health.

Key Herbs for Lupus

1. **Turmeric (Curcuma longa)**:
    - **Properties**: Anti-inflammatory and antioxidant.
    - **Usage**: Can be added to foods, taken as a supplement, or consumed as tea to help manage inflammation and support overall health.

2. **Ginger (Zingiber officinale)**:
    - **Properties**: Anti-inflammatory and may help reduce pain and swelling.
    - **Usage**: Consumed as tea, added to meals, or taken as a supplement.

3. **Boswellia (Boswellia serrata)**:
    - **Properties**: Anti-inflammatory, helps with joint pain and inflammation.
    - **Usage**: Taken as a supplement to help manage inflammation associated with lupus.

4. **Green Tea (Camellia sinensis)**:
    - **Properties**: Antioxidant, supports immune system health.
    - **Usage**: Consumed as tea or in supplement form to support overall health and reduce oxidative stress.

5. **Ashwagandha (Withania somnifera)**:
    - **Properties**: Adaptogenic herb that may help with stress management and support immune function.
    - **Usage**: Taken as a supplement to help manage stress and support overall well-being.

6. **Milk Thistle (Silybum marianum)**:
    - **Properties**: Supports liver health and detoxification.

- **Usage**: Taken as a supplement to support liver function and overall detoxification.

Dietary Recommendations for Lupus

1. **Anti-Inflammatory Diet**:
   - **Purpose**: Reduces inflammation and supports overall health.
   - **Include**:
     - **Fruits and Vegetables**: Berries, leafy greens, and cruciferous vegetables.
     - **Fatty Fish**: Salmon, mackerel, and sardines.
     - **Nuts and Seeds**: Walnuts, flaxseeds, and chia seeds.

2. **Omega-3 Fatty Acids**:
   - **Importance**: Helps reduce inflammation and support cardiovascular health.
   - **Include**: Fatty fish, flaxseeds, chia seeds, and walnuts.

3. **Avoid Processed Foods**:
   - **Reason**: Processed foods can exacerbate inflammation and contribute to poor health.
   - **Recommendation**: Limit or avoid processed and sugary foods.

4. **Gluten-Free Diet**:
   - **Purpose**: Some individuals with lupus may benefit from avoiding gluten.
   - **Include**: Gluten-free grains like quinoa, rice, and millet.

5. **Hydration**:
   - **Importance**: Supports overall health and helps manage symptoms.
   - **Guideline**: Drink plenty of water throughout the day and avoid excessive caffeine and alcohol.

6. **Balanced Protein Intake**:
   - **Purpose**: Supports muscle health and immune function.
   - **Include**: Lean proteins such as poultry, fish, and plant-based proteins like beans and lentils.

7. **Limit Saturated and Trans Fats**:
   - **Reason**: These fats can exacerbate inflammation.

- **Recommendation**: Opt for healthy fats from sources like avocados, nuts, and olive oil.

Lifestyle Changes

1. **Stress Management**:
   - **Importance**: Stress can trigger or worsen lupus symptoms.
   - **Techniques**: Practice relaxation techniques like deep breathing, meditation, and yoga.

2. **Regular Exercise**:
   - **Benefits**: Helps manage symptoms, improves overall health, and reduces fatigue.
   - **Examples**: Low-impact exercises such as walking, swimming, or cycling.

3. **Adequate Rest**:
   - **Purpose**: Supports overall health and helps manage fatigue.
   - **Guideline**: Aim for 7-9 hours of quality sleep each night and incorporate rest periods during the day if needed.

4. **Sun Protection**:
   - **Importance**: Sun exposure can exacerbate lupus symptoms.
   - **Guideline**: Use sunscreen, wear protective clothing, and avoid prolonged sun exposure.

5. **Avoid Smoking and Limit Alcohol**:
   - **Reason**: Smoking and excessive alcohol can worsen lupus symptoms and overall health.
   - **Guideline**: Avoid smoking and limit alcohol intake.

Additional Therapies

1. **Acupuncture**:
   - **Benefits**: May help with pain management and inflammation reduction.

2. **Massage Therapy**:
   - **Usage**: Can help alleviate muscle and joint pain associated with lupus.

3. **Mindfulness and Cognitive Behavioral Therapy (CBT)**:

- **Purpose**: Supports mental health, helps manage stress, and improves coping strategies.

4. **Supplements**:
   - **Vitamin D**: Supports immune function and overall health.
   - **Probiotics**: Supports gut health and may help manage inflammation.

Conclusion

Managing lupus holistically involves a comprehensive approach that includes dietary adjustments, herbal remedies, lifestyle changes, and supportive therapies. By incorporating these strategies, you can help reduce inflammation, manage symptoms, and support overall health. Always consult with a healthcare provider before starting any new treatment plan or making significant changes to your current regimen.

Lyme Disease

Lyme Disease is a tick-borne illness caused by the bacterium *Borrelia burgdorferi*. It can lead to a variety of symptoms, including fever, fatigue, headache, and a characteristic "bull's-eye" rash. Chronic Lyme Disease may involve more complex symptoms affecting the joints, heart, and nervous system. Managing Lyme Disease holistically involves using herbal remedies, dietary adjustments, lifestyle changes, and supportive therapies to help reduce symptoms, support the immune system, and promote overall health.

Key Herbs for Lyme Disease

1. **Cat's Claw (Uncaria tomentosa)**:
   - **Properties**: Immune-modulating, anti-inflammatory.
   - **Usage**: Taken as a supplement or in tea to support immune function and reduce inflammation.

2. **Japanese Knotweed (Fallopia japonica)**:
   - **Properties**: Rich in resveratrol, supports immune health and helps with inflammation.
   - **Usage**: Consumed as a supplement to support immune function and manage symptoms.

3. **Andrographis (Andrographis paniculata)**:
   - **Properties**: Antimicrobial, supports the immune system.
   - **Usage**: Taken as a supplement to help manage infection and support immune health.

4. **Garlic (Allium sativum)**:
   - **Properties**: Antimicrobial, supports immune function.
   - **Usage**: Added to foods or taken as a supplement to help fight infections and support overall health.

5. **Echinacea (Echinacea spp.)**:
   - **Properties**: Immune-boosting, helps with infection control.
   - **Usage**: Consumed as tea or in supplement form to support the immune system.

6. **Turmeric (Curcuma longa)**:
   - **Properties**: Anti-inflammatory, supports joint and immune health.
   - **Usage**: Added to foods, taken as a supplement, or consumed as tea.

Dietary Recommendations for Lyme Disease

1. **Anti-Inflammatory Diet**:
   - **Purpose**: Reduces inflammation and supports overall health.
   - **Include**:
     - **Fruits and Vegetables**: Berries, leafy greens, and cruciferous vegetables.
     - **Fatty Fish**: Salmon, mackerel, and sardines.
     - **Nuts and Seeds**: Walnuts, flaxseeds, and chia seeds.

2. **High Antioxidant Foods**:
   - **Importance**: Supports overall health and helps combat oxidative stress.
   - **Include**:
     - **Berries**: Blueberries, strawberries, and raspberries.
     - **Leafy Greens**: Spinach, kale, and Swiss chard.

3. **Gluten-Free Diet**:
   - **Purpose**: Some individuals with Lyme Disease may benefit from avoiding gluten.
   - **Include**: Gluten-free grains like quinoa, rice, and millet.

4. **Hydration**:

- **Importance**: Supports detoxification and overall health.
- **Guideline**: Drink plenty of water throughout the day and avoid excessive caffeine and alcohol.

5. **Supportive Supplements**:
    - **Vitamin C**: Supports immune function and overall health.
    - **Vitamin D**: Important for immune system health.
    - **Probiotics**: Supports gut health and overall well-being.

6. **Avoid Processed Foods and Sugar**:
    - **Reason**: Processed foods and sugar can exacerbate inflammation.
    - **Recommendation**: Limit or avoid processed foods and sugary snacks.

Lifestyle Changes

1. **Stress Management**:
    - **Importance**: Stress can worsen symptoms and affect overall health.
    - **Techniques**: Practice relaxation techniques like deep breathing, meditation, and yoga.

2. **Regular Exercise**:
    - **Benefits**: Helps manage symptoms, improves overall health, and reduces fatigue.
    - **Examples**: Low-impact exercises such as walking, swimming, or cycling.

3. **Adequate Rest**:
    - **Purpose**: Supports overall health and helps manage fatigue.
    - **Guideline**: Aim for 7-9 hours of quality sleep each night and incorporate rest periods during the day if needed.

4. **Tick Prevention**:
    - **Importance**: Reduces the risk of re-infection.
    - **Guideline**: Use tick repellents, wear protective clothing, and check for ticks after spending time outdoors.

5. **Detoxification**:
    - **Purpose**: Supports the body's natural detoxification processes.

- **Methods**: Include practices such as drinking plenty of water, consuming detoxifying foods (e.g., cilantro, garlic), and engaging in regular physical activity.

Additional Therapies

1. **Acupuncture**:
   - **Benefits**: May help with pain management and overall symptom relief.

2. **Massage Therapy**:
   - **Usage**: Can help alleviate muscle and joint pain associated with Lyme Disease.

3. **Biofeedback**:
   - **Purpose**: Helps manage stress and physiological responses that affect health.

4. **Ozone Therapy**:
   - **Benefits**: May support detoxification and overall health in some individuals.

5. **Chelation Therapy**:
   - **Purpose**: Supports detoxification, particularly in cases of heavy metal exposure.

Conclusion

Managing Lyme Disease holistically involves a multi-faceted approach that includes dietary adjustments, herbal remedies, lifestyle changes, and supportive therapies. By incorporating these strategies, you can help reduce symptoms, support the immune system, and promote overall health. Always consult with a healthcare provider before starting any new treatment plan or making significant changes to your current regimen.

Multiple Sclerosis

Multiple Sclerosis (MS) is a chronic autoimmune disease that affects the central nervous system (CNS), leading to the deterioration or permanent damage to myelin, the protective covering of nerve fibers. Symptoms can vary widely and may include fatigue, muscle weakness, difficulty with coordination, vision problems, and cognitive changes. Managing MS holistically involves using a combination of dietary adjustments, herbal remedies, lifestyle changes, and supportive therapies to help manage symptoms, support overall health, and improve quality of life.

Key Herbs for Multiple Sclerosis

1. **Turmeric (Curcuma longa)**:

- **Properties**: Anti-inflammatory, antioxidant.
- **Usage**: Can be added to foods, taken as a supplement, or consumed as tea to help manage inflammation and support overall health.

2. **Ginger (Zingiber officinale)**:
   - **Properties**: Anti-inflammatory, helps reduce pain and muscle spasticity.
   - **Usage**: Consumed as tea, added to meals, or taken as a supplement.

3. **Bacopa (Bacopa monnieri)**:
   - **Properties**: Supports cognitive function and reduces stress.
   - **Usage**: Taken as a supplement to help support cognitive health and manage stress.

4. **Gingko Biloba (Gingko biloba)**:
   - **Properties**: Enhances cognitive function and improves circulation.
   - **Usage**: Taken as a supplement to support cognitive health and improve circulation.

5. **Ashwagandha (Withania somnifera)**:
   - **Properties**: Adaptogenic herb that may help with stress management and overall well-being.
   - **Usage**: Taken as a supplement to help manage stress and support overall health.

6. **Evening Primrose Oil (Oenothera biennis)**:
   - **Properties**: Contains gamma-linolenic acid (GLA), which may help reduce inflammation.
   - **Usage**: Taken as a supplement to support overall health and manage inflammation.

Dietary Recommendations for Multiple Sclerosis

1. **Anti-Inflammatory Diet**:
   - **Purpose**: Reduces inflammation and supports overall health.
   - **Include**:
     - **Fruits and Vegetables**: Berries, leafy greens, and cruciferous vegetables.
     - **Fatty Fish**: Salmon, mackerel, and sardines.

- **Nuts and Seeds**: Walnuts, flaxseeds, and chia seeds.
2. **Omega-3 Fatty Acids**:
    - **Importance**: Helps reduce inflammation and support brain health.
    - **Include**: Fatty fish, flaxseeds, chia seeds, and walnuts.
3. **Low-FODMAP Diet**:
    - **Purpose**: May help manage digestive symptoms that can accompany MS.
    - **Include**:
        - **Low-FODMAP Foods**: Carrots, spinach, and rice.
        - **Avoid**: High-FODMAP foods like onions, garlic, and apples.
4. **Gluten-Free Diet**:
    - **Purpose**: Some individuals with MS may benefit from avoiding gluten.
    - **Include**: Gluten-free grains like quinoa, rice, and millet.
5. **Hydration**:
    - **Importance**: Supports overall health and helps manage symptoms.
    - **Guideline**: Drink plenty of water throughout the day and avoid excessive caffeine and alcohol.
6. **Vitamin D**:
    - **Importance**: Supports immune function and may help manage MS symptoms.
    - **Include**: Vitamin D-rich foods like fatty fish, fortified dairy, and mushrooms, or consider supplements if recommended by a healthcare provider.
7. **Balanced Protein Intake**:
    - **Purpose**: Supports muscle health and overall well-being.
    - **Include**: Lean proteins such as poultry, fish, and plant-based proteins like beans and lentils.
8. **Avoid Processed Foods and Sugar**:
    - **Reason**: Processed foods and sugar can exacerbate inflammation.
    - **Recommendation**: Limit or avoid processed foods and sugary snacks.

Lifestyle Changes

1. **Stress Management**:
   - **Importance**: Stress can exacerbate MS symptoms.
   - **Techniques**: Practice relaxation techniques like deep breathing, meditation, and yoga.

2. **Regular Exercise**:
   - **Benefits**: Helps manage symptoms, improves overall health, and reduces fatigue.
   - **Examples**: Low-impact exercises such as swimming, walking, or stationary cycling.

3. **Adequate Rest**:
   - **Purpose**: Supports overall health and helps manage fatigue.
   - **Guideline**: Aim for 7-9 hours of quality sleep each night and incorporate rest periods during the day if needed.

4. **Cognitive and Physical Therapy**:
   - **Importance**: Helps with symptom management and improves quality of life.
   - **Types**: Engage in physical therapy for mobility and strength, and cognitive therapy for mental functioning.

5. **Avoid Overheating**:
   - **Reason**: Heat can exacerbate MS symptoms in some individuals.
   - **Guideline**: Use cooling techniques and avoid hot environments.

6. **Support Groups**:
   - **Purpose**: Provides emotional support and practical advice.
   - **Recommendation**: Join MS support groups or communities for shared experiences and support.

Additional Therapies

1. **Acupuncture**:
   - **Benefits**: May help with pain management, muscle spasticity, and overall symptom relief.

2. **Massage Therapy**:
   - **Usage**: Can help alleviate muscle tension and improve relaxation.

3. **Biofeedback**:
    - **Purpose**: Helps manage stress and physiological responses that affect health.
4. **Reiki or Energy Healing**:
    - **Benefits**: May support relaxation and overall well-being.
5. **Naturopathic Medicine**:
    - **Purpose**: Offers a holistic approach to managing symptoms and supporting overall health.

Conclusion

Managing Multiple Sclerosis holistically involves a comprehensive approach that includes dietary adjustments, herbal remedies, lifestyle changes, and supportive therapies. By incorporating these strategies, you can help manage symptoms, reduce inflammation, support overall health, and improve quality of life. Always consult with a healthcare provider before starting any new treatment plan or making significant changes to your current regimen.

Adrenal Fatigue

Adrenal Fatigue is a term used to describe a collection of symptoms believed to be caused by the overuse and subsequent exhaustion of the adrenal glands, which are responsible for producing hormones like cortisol that help manage stress. Symptoms can include chronic fatigue, difficulty sleeping, weight gain, and trouble handling stress. Managing adrenal fatigue holistically involves a combination of dietary adjustments, herbal remedies, lifestyle changes, and supportive therapies to restore adrenal function, balance hormones, and improve overall well-being.

Key Herbs for Adrenal Fatigue

1. **Ashwagandha (Withania somnifera)**:
    - **Properties**: Adaptogenic herb that helps the body cope with stress and supports adrenal health.
    - **Usage**: Taken as a supplement to help balance cortisol levels and improve resilience to stress.
2. **Rhodiola (Rhodiola rosea)**:
    - **Properties**: Adaptogen that supports energy levels, reduces fatigue, and enhances mental performance.
    - **Usage**: Taken as a supplement to boost energy and manage stress.

3. **Holy Basil (Ocimum sanctum)**:
    - **Properties**: Adaptogenic herb that helps regulate stress hormones and supports overall well-being.
    - **Usage**: Consumed as tea or in supplement form to help balance stress and support adrenal function.

4. **Licorice Root (Glycyrrhiza glabra)**:
    - **Properties**: Supports adrenal function and helps maintain cortisol levels.
    - **Usage**: Taken as a supplement or in tea; use with caution as it can affect blood pressure and electrolyte balance.

5. **Ginseng (Panax ginseng)**:
    - **Properties**: Enhances energy, reduces fatigue, and supports adrenal health.
    - **Usage**: Taken as a supplement to support energy levels and manage stress.

6. **Siberian Ginseng (Eleutherococcus senticosus)**:
    - **Properties**: Adaptogen that improves endurance and helps manage stress.
    - **Usage**: Consumed as a supplement to support adrenal function and increase energy.

Dietary Recommendations for Adrenal Fatigue

1. **Balanced Diet**:
    - **Purpose**: Provides essential nutrients to support adrenal health and overall energy levels.
    - **Include**:
        - **Whole Foods**: Fresh fruits, vegetables, lean proteins, and whole grains.
        - **Healthy Fats**: Avocados, nuts, seeds, and olive oil.

2. **Regular, Balanced Meals**:
    - **Importance**: Stabilizes blood sugar levels and prevents energy crashes.
    - **Include**:
        - **Protein**: Helps maintain stable energy levels.
        - **Complex Carbohydrates**: Provide sustained energy.

3. **Reduce Caffeine Intake**:

- **Reason**: Excessive caffeine can stress the adrenal glands and disrupt sleep.
- **Recommendation**: Limit caffeine and consider switching to herbal teas like chamomile or rooibos.

4. **Avoid Sugar and Processed Foods**:
   - **Reason**: Sugar and processed foods can cause blood sugar imbalances and stress the adrenal glands.
   - **Recommendation**: Focus on whole, unprocessed foods and limit sugary snacks.

5. **Hydration**:
   - **Importance**: Supports overall health and adrenal function.
   - **Guideline**: Drink plenty of water throughout the day and consider adding electrolyte-rich beverages like coconut water.

6. **Supportive Supplements**:
   - **Vitamin C**: Supports adrenal function and helps manage stress.
   - **B Vitamins**: Important for energy production and stress management.
   - **Magnesium**: Helps relax muscles and support adrenal function.

Lifestyle Changes

1. **Stress Management**:
   - **Importance**: Reduces the load on the adrenal glands and improves overall well-being.
   - **Techniques**: Practice relaxation techniques like deep breathing, meditation, and yoga.

2. **Regular Exercise**:
   - **Benefits**: Helps manage stress, supports energy levels, and improves overall health.
   - **Examples**: Low to moderate exercise such as walking, swimming, or gentle yoga.

3. **Adequate Sleep**:
   - **Purpose**: Supports adrenal recovery and overall health.
   - **Guideline**: Aim for 7-9 hours of quality sleep each night and establish a consistent sleep routine.

4. **Avoid Overworking and Burnout**:
   - **Reason**: Excessive work and stress can exacerbate adrenal fatigue.
   - **Guideline**: Prioritize work-life balance and take breaks to prevent burnout.

5. **Mindfulness and Relaxation Techniques**:
   - **Purpose**: Supports stress management and adrenal health.
   - **Techniques**: Engage in activities like mindfulness meditation, deep breathing exercises, and progressive muscle relaxation.

6. **Healthy Relationships and Social Support**:
   - **Importance**: Provides emotional support and helps manage stress.
   - **Recommendation**: Connect with supportive friends, family, or support groups.

Additional Therapies

1. **Acupuncture**:
   - **Benefits**: May help with stress reduction and overall adrenal support.

2. **Massage Therapy**:
   - **Usage**: Can help alleviate tension and support relaxation.

3. **Biofeedback**:
   - **Purpose**: Helps manage stress and physiological responses.

4. **Reiki or Energy Healing**:
   - **Benefits**: Supports relaxation and overall well-being.

5. **Naturopathic Medicine**:
   - **Purpose**: Offers a holistic approach to managing symptoms and supporting adrenal health.

Conclusion

Managing adrenal fatigue holistically involves a comprehensive approach that includes dietary adjustments, herbal remedies, lifestyle changes, and supportive therapies. By incorporating these strategies, you can help restore adrenal function, balance hormones, and improve overall well-being. Always consult with a healthcare provider before starting any new treatment plan or making significant changes to your current regimen.

Parasites

Parasitic infections occur when organisms such as protozoa, helminths, or ectoparasites invade the body and cause symptoms ranging from mild discomfort to severe illness. Common symptoms of parasitic infections include digestive disturbances, fatigue, weight loss, and skin issues. Managing parasitic infections holistically involves using a combination of herbal remedies, dietary adjustments, lifestyle changes, and supportive therapies to eliminate parasites, restore health, and support overall well-being.

Key Herbs for Parasites

1. **Wormwood (Artemisia absinthium)**:
   - **Properties**: Antimicrobial, antiparasitic.
   - **Usage**: Taken as a supplement or in tea to help eliminate parasites and support digestive health.

2. **Black Walnut (Juglans nigra)**:
   - **Properties**: Antimicrobial, antiparasitic.
   - **Usage**: Consumed as a tincture or supplement to help manage parasitic infections.

3. **Cloves (Syzygium aromaticum)**:
   - **Properties**: Antimicrobial, antiparasitic.
   - **Usage**: Used in food or taken as a supplement to help eliminate parasites and support overall health.

4. **Garlic (Allium sativum)**:
   - **Properties**: Antimicrobial, antiparasitic.
   - **Usage**: Added to foods or taken as a supplement to help fight infections and support overall health.

5. **Neem (Azadirachta indica)**:
   - **Properties**: Antimicrobial, antiparasitic.
   - **Usage**: Consumed as a supplement or in tea to help eliminate parasites and support immune health.

6. **Papaya Seeds (Carica papaya)**:
   - **Properties**: Antiparasitic, digestive aid.

- **Usage**: Consumed as a food or supplement to help with parasite elimination and digestive health.

Dietary Recommendations for Parasites

1. **Anti-Parasitic Foods**:
   - **Purpose**: Supports the elimination of parasites and supports overall health.
   - **Include**:
     - **Pumpkin Seeds**: Contains compounds that may help eliminate parasites.
     - **Pineapple**: Contains bromelain, which may help digest parasites and support overall health.

2. **Fiber-Rich Foods**:
   - **Importance**: Helps with detoxification and digestive health.
   - **Include**:
     - **Vegetables**: Leafy greens, carrots, and beets.
     - **Fruits**: Apples, pears, and berries.

3. **Probiotic Foods**:
   - **Purpose**: Supports gut health and helps restore balance after a parasitic infection.
   - **Include**:
     - **Fermented Foods**: Yogurt, kefir, sauerkraut, and kimchi.

4. **Avoid Sugar and Processed Foods**:
   - **Reason**: Sugar and processed foods can support parasitic growth and weaken the immune system.
   - **Recommendation**: Focus on whole, unprocessed foods and limit sugary snacks.

5. **Hydration**:
   - **Importance**: Supports overall health and helps with detoxification.
   - **Guideline**: Drink plenty of water throughout the day and consider adding detoxifying beverages like herbal teas.

6. **Anti-Inflammatory Diet**:

- **Purpose**: Reduces inflammation and supports overall health.
- **Include**:
  - **Fruits and Vegetables**: Berries, leafy greens, and cruciferous vegetables.
  - **Healthy Fats**: Avocados, nuts, seeds, and olive oil.

Lifestyle Changes

1. **Proper Hygiene**:
   - **Importance**: Reduces the risk of parasitic infections.
   - **Guideline**: Practice good handwashing, especially before eating and after using the restroom.

2. **Safe Food Preparation**:
   - **Purpose**: Prevents parasitic infections from contaminated food.
   - **Guideline**: Ensure thorough cooking of meats, wash fruits and vegetables, and avoid eating raw or undercooked foods.

3. **Regular Detoxification**:
   - **Importance**: Supports the body's natural elimination of parasites.
   - **Methods**: Engage in regular detox programs that include hydration, herbal teas, and dietary adjustments.

4. **Avoid Contaminated Water**:
   - **Reason**: Contaminated water can be a source of parasitic infections.
   - **Guideline**: Drink clean, filtered water and avoid consuming water from uncertain sources.

5. **Regular Exercise**:
   - **Benefits**: Supports overall health and boosts immune function.
   - **Examples**: Engage in regular physical activity such as walking, swimming, or cycling.

6. **Health Monitoring**:
   - **Purpose**: Detects potential parasitic infections early.
   - **Guideline**: Regularly monitor for symptoms and seek medical advice if necessary.

Additional Therapies

1. **Acupuncture**:
   - **Benefits**: May help with symptom management and overall health support.

2. **Massage Therapy**:
   - **Usage**: Can help alleviate discomfort and support overall well-being.

3. **Biofeedback**:
   - **Purpose**: Helps manage stress and physiological responses.

4. **Reiki or Energy Healing**:
   - **Benefits**: Supports relaxation and overall well-being.

5. **Naturopathic Medicine**:
   - **Purpose**: Offers a holistic approach to managing symptoms and supporting overall health.

Conclusion

Managing parasitic infections holistically involves a multi-faceted approach that includes dietary adjustments, herbal remedies, lifestyle changes, and supportive therapies. By incorporating these strategies, you can help eliminate parasites, support overall health, and improve well-being. Always consult with a healthcare provider before starting any new treatment plan or making significant changes to your current regimen.

Candida Overgrowth

Candida overgrowth occurs when the yeast-like fungus Candida albicans proliferates beyond its normal levels, leading to various symptoms. Candida is normally present in small amounts in the body, but an overgrowth can cause issues such as digestive disturbances, fatigue, recurrent infections, and skin problems. Managing Candida overgrowth holistically involves using dietary adjustments, herbal remedies, lifestyle changes, and supportive therapies to restore balance and improve overall health.

Key Herbs for Candida Overgrowth

1. **Garlic (Allium sativum)**:
   - **Properties**: Antifungal, antimicrobial.
   - **Usage**: Consumed raw, added to food, or taken as a supplement to help combat Candida and support immune health.

2. **Oregano Oil (Origanum vulgare)**:

- o **Properties**: Potent antifungal.
- o **Usage**: Taken as a supplement or diluted in water for topical application to help manage Candida overgrowth.

3. **Pau d'Arco (Tabebuia impetiginosa)**:
   - o **Properties**: Antifungal, antimicrobial.
   - o **Usage**: Consumed as tea or taken as a supplement to help address Candida and support overall health.

4. **Coconut Oil (Cocos nucifera)**:
   - o **Properties**: Contains caprylic acid, which has antifungal properties.
   - o **Usage**: Consumed as part of the diet or used topically to help manage Candida overgrowth.

5. **Grapefruit Seed Extract (Citrus paradisi)**:
   - o **Properties**: Antifungal, antimicrobial.
   - o **Usage**: Taken as a supplement to help combat Candida and support overall health.

6. **Echinacea (Echinacea purpurea)**:
   - o **Properties**: Supports immune function.
   - o **Usage**: Taken as a supplement or in tea to help support the body's defenses against Candida overgrowth.

Dietary Recommendations for Candida Overgrowth

1. **Low-Sugar Diet**:
   - o **Purpose**: Reduces food sources for Candida.
   - o **Include**:
     - **Non-Starchy Vegetables**: Leafy greens, cucumbers, and bell peppers.
     - **Lean Proteins**: Chicken, turkey, and fish.
     - **Healthy Fats**: Avocados, nuts, and olive oil.

2. **Anti-Candida Foods**:
   - o **Purpose**: Supports the reduction of Candida overgrowth.
   - o **Include**:
     - **Garlic and Onions**: Known for their antifungal properties.

- **Fermented Foods**: Sauerkraut, kimchi, and kefir to support gut health.

3. **Avoid Processed Foods and Sugar**:
    - **Reason**: Sugar and processed foods can fuel Candida growth.
    - **Recommendation**: Focus on whole, unprocessed foods and avoid sugary snacks and beverages.

4. **Incorporate Probiotics**:
    - **Purpose**: Supports a healthy balance of gut microbiota.
    - **Include**:
        - **Probiotic Foods**: Yogurt, kefir, and fermented vegetables.

5. **Hydration**:
    - **Importance**: Supports detoxification and overall health.
    - **Guideline**: Drink plenty of water throughout the day and consider herbal teas with antifungal properties.

6. **Balanced Nutrients**:
    - **Purpose**: Supports overall health and immune function.
    - **Include**:
        - **Whole Grains**: Brown rice, quinoa, and oats.
        - **Lean Proteins**: Eggs, tofu, and legumes.

Lifestyle Changes

1. **Reduce Stress**:
    - **Importance**: Stress can weaken the immune system and exacerbate Candida overgrowth.
    - **Techniques**: Practice relaxation techniques like deep breathing, meditation, and yoga.

2. **Regular Exercise**:
    - **Benefits**: Supports overall health and immune function.
    - **Examples**: Engage in regular physical activity such as walking, swimming, or cycling.

3. **Adequate Sleep**:

- **Purpose**: Supports immune function and overall health.
- **Guideline**: Aim for 7-9 hours of quality sleep each night and establish a consistent sleep routine.

4. **Avoid Antibiotics When Possible**:
    - **Reason**: Antibiotics can disrupt the balance of gut microbiota and contribute to Candida overgrowth.
    - **Guideline**: Use antibiotics only when necessary and prescribed by a healthcare provider.

5. **Healthy Hygiene Practices**:
    - **Purpose**: Reduces the risk of infections and supports overall health.
    - **Guideline**: Practice good personal hygiene, including regular handwashing and avoiding sharing personal items.

6. **Support Gut Health**:
    - **Importance**: A healthy gut microbiome supports balance and reduces Candida overgrowth.
    - **Techniques**: Incorporate prebiotics and probiotics into your diet to support gut health.

Additional Therapies

1. **Acupuncture**:
    - **Benefits**: May help with symptom management and overall health support.

2. **Massage Therapy**:
    - **Usage**: Can help alleviate discomfort and support overall well-being.

3. **Biofeedback**:
    - **Purpose**: Helps manage stress and physiological responses.

4. **Reiki or Energy Healing**:
    - **Benefits**: Supports relaxation and overall well-being.

5. **Naturopathic Medicine**:
    - **Purpose**: Offers a holistic approach to managing symptoms and supporting overall health.

Conclusion

Managing Candida overgrowth holistically involves a comprehensive approach that includes dietary adjustments, herbal remedies, lifestyle changes, and supportive therapies. By incorporating these strategies, you can help restore balance, support immune health, and improve overall well-being. Always consult with a healthcare provider before starting any new treatment plan or making significant changes to your current regimen.

Anti-Aging Strategies

Anti-aging strategies aim to slow down the aging process, promote longevity, and enhance overall health and vitality. A holistic approach to anti-aging involves using dietary adjustments, herbal remedies, lifestyle changes, and supportive therapies to maintain youthful function, improve skin health, and support overall well-being.

Key Herbs for Anti-Aging

1. **Ginseng (Panax ginseng)**:
    - **Properties**: Antioxidant, adaptogen.
    - **Usage**: Taken as a supplement or tea to boost energy, support mental function, and combat signs of aging.

2. **Turmeric (Curcuma longa)**:
    - **Properties**: Anti-inflammatory, antioxidant.
    - **Usage**: Consumed as a spice in foods or taken as a supplement to support joint health, skin health, and overall vitality.

3. **Green Tea (Camellia sinensis)**:
    - **Properties**: Antioxidant, anti-inflammatory.
    - **Usage**: Consumed as tea or in supplement form to support skin health, protect against oxidative damage, and improve metabolism.

4. **Gotu Kola (Centella asiatica)**:
    - **Properties**: Antioxidant, skin rejuvenation.
    - **Usage**: Taken as a supplement or used topically to support skin health, improve circulation, and enhance cognitive function.

5. **Reishi Mushroom (Ganoderma lucidum)**:
    - **Properties**: Immune-supportive, antioxidant.
    - **Usage**: Taken as a supplement or in tea to boost immune function, support stress management, and promote longevity.

6. **Hawthorn Berry (Crataegus spp.)**:
   - **Properties**: Antioxidant, cardiovascular support.
   - **Usage**: Consumed as a supplement or in tea to support heart health and improve circulation.

Dietary Recommendations for Anti-Aging

1. **Antioxidant-Rich Foods**:
   - **Purpose**: Protects cells from oxidative damage and supports overall health.
   - **Include**:
     - **Berries**: Blueberries, strawberries, and raspberries.
     - **Nuts and Seeds**: Almonds, walnuts, and flaxseeds.
     - **Vegetables**: Spinach, kale, and bell peppers.

2. **Healthy Fats**:
   - **Importance**: Supports skin health and cognitive function.
   - **Include**:
     - **Avocados**: Rich in healthy fats and vitamins.
     - **Olive Oil**: Contains antioxidants and healthy fats.
     - **Fatty Fish**: Salmon, mackerel, and sardines.

3. **Hydrating Foods**:
   - **Purpose**: Maintains skin hydration and overall health.
   - **Include**:
     - **Watermelon**: High water content and antioxidants.
     - **Cucumbers**: Hydrating and low in calories.
     - **Celery**: Supports hydration and provides essential nutrients.

4. **Lean Proteins**:
   - **Importance**: Supports muscle health and repair.
   - **Include**:
     - **Chicken**: Lean protein source.
     - **Tofu**: Plant-based protein.

- **Legumes**: Beans, lentils, and chickpeas.

5. **Whole Grains**:
    - **Purpose**: Provides sustained energy and supports digestive health.
    - **Include**:
        - **Quinoa**: High in protein and nutrients.
        - **Brown Rice**: Provides fiber and essential minerals.
        - **Oats**: Supports heart health and digestion.

6. **Limit Processed Foods and Sugar**:
    - **Reason**: Reduces inflammation and oxidative stress.
    - **Recommendation**: Focus on whole, unprocessed foods and limit sugary snacks and beverages.

Lifestyle Changes for Anti-Aging

1. **Regular Exercise**:
    - **Benefits**: Supports cardiovascular health, muscle tone, and overall vitality.
    - **Examples**: Engage in activities such as walking, swimming, or strength training.

2. **Adequate Sleep**:
    - **Purpose**: Supports cellular repair and overall health.
    - **Guideline**: Aim for 7-9 hours of quality sleep each night and maintain a consistent sleep schedule.

3. **Stress Management**:
    - **Importance**: Reduces the impact of stress on the body and slows the aging process.
    - **Techniques**: Practice relaxation techniques such as mindfulness, deep breathing, and yoga.

4. **Hydration**:
    - **Importance**: Maintains skin elasticity and overall health.
    - **Guideline**: Drink plenty of water throughout the day and consider adding herbal teas for additional benefits.

5. **Skin Care**:

- **Purpose**: Supports skin health and reduces signs of aging.
- **Routine**: Use gentle cleansers, moisturizers, and sunscreen to protect and rejuvenate the skin.

6. **Mental Stimulation**:
    - **Benefits**: Supports cognitive function and mental health.
    - **Activities**: Engage in activities such as reading, puzzles, and learning new skills.

Additional Therapies

1. **Acupuncture**:
    - **Benefits**: May help with stress reduction, energy balance, and overall well-being.

2. **Massage Therapy**:
    - **Usage**: Can help with relaxation, improve circulation, and support overall health.

3. **Biofeedback**:
    - **Purpose**: Helps manage stress and physiological responses.

4. **Reiki or Energy Healing**:
    - **Benefits**: Supports relaxation and overall well-being.

5. **Naturopathic Medicine**:
    - **Purpose**: Offers a holistic approach to managing aging and supporting overall health.

Conclusion

Implementing anti-aging strategies holistically involves a multi-faceted approach that includes dietary adjustments, herbal remedies, lifestyle changes, and supportive therapies. By incorporating these practices into your daily routine, you can support overall health, enhance vitality, and promote a youthful appearance. Always consult with a healthcare provider before starting any new treatment plan or making significant changes to your current regimen.

Flu, Viral, and Immune System Support

Supporting the immune system and managing symptoms of flu and viral infections involves a comprehensive approach that includes dietary adjustments, herbal remedies, lifestyle changes, and supportive therapies. A strong immune system helps the body fight off infections and recover more quickly from illnesses.

Key Herbs for Immune Support and Viral Infections

1. **Echinacea (Echinacea purpurea)**:
    - **Properties**: Immune-stimulant, antiviral.
    - **Usage**: Taken as a supplement or in tea to help boost the immune system and reduce the severity and duration of viral infections.

2. **Elderberry (Sambucus nigra)**:
    - **Properties**: Antiviral, immune-supportive.
    - **Usage**: Consumed as a syrup or supplement to help manage symptoms of flu and colds and support immune health.

3. **Ginger (Zingiber officinale)**:
    - **Properties**: Anti-inflammatory, antiviral.
    - **Usage**: Used in tea or added to foods to support the immune system and help relieve symptoms of colds and flu.

4. **Garlic (Allium sativum)**:
    - **Properties**: Antimicrobial, immune-boosting.
    - **Usage**: Consumed raw, added to food, or taken as a supplement to enhance immune function and fight infections.

5. **Astragalus (Astragalus membranaceus)**:
    - **Properties**: Immune-supportive, adaptogen.
    - **Usage**: Taken as a supplement or in tea to support immune health and help the body adapt to stress.

6. **Licorice Root (Glycyrrhiza glabra)**:
    - **Properties**: Anti-inflammatory, immune-supportive.
    - **Usage**: Consumed as tea or in supplement form to support respiratory health and overall immune function.

Dietary Recommendations for Immune Support

1. **Vitamin C-Rich Foods**:
    - **Purpose**: Supports immune function and helps combat infections.

- Include:
    - **Citrus Fruits**: Oranges, grapefruits, and lemons.
    - **Berries**: Strawberries, blueberries, and raspberries.
    - **Vegetables**: Bell peppers, broccoli, and Brussels sprouts.

2. **Vitamin D-Rich Foods**:
    - **Importance**: Supports immune function and reduces the risk of infections.
    - Include:
        - **Fatty Fish**: Salmon, mackerel, and sardines.
        - **Fortified Foods**: Fortified milk, orange juice, and cereals.
        - **Eggs**: Provide vitamin D and other essential nutrients.

3. **Zinc-Rich Foods**:
    - **Purpose**: Supports immune function and helps the body fight off infections.
    - Include:
        - **Nuts and Seeds**: Pumpkin seeds, cashews, and sunflower seeds.
        - **Lean Meats**: Beef, pork, and chicken.
        - **Legumes**: Lentils, chickpeas, and beans.

4. **Probiotic Foods**:
    - **Importance**: Supports gut health, which is closely linked to immune function.
    - Include:
        - **Yogurt**: Contains beneficial bacteria to support gut health.
        - **Kefir**: Fermented dairy with probiotics.
        - **Fermented Vegetables**: Sauerkraut, kimchi, and pickles.

5. **Hydrating Foods**:
    - **Purpose**: Supports overall health and helps the body recover from infections.
    - Include:
        - **Soups and Broths**: Provide hydration and nutrients.
        - **Watermelon**: High water content and vitamins.

- **Cucumbers**: Hydrating and low in calories.
6. **Anti-Inflammatory Foods**:
    - **Importance**: Reduces inflammation and supports immune health.
    - **Include**:
        - **Turmeric**: Contains curcumin, which has anti-inflammatory properties.
        - **Green Tea**: Rich in antioxidants and anti-inflammatory compounds.
        - **Olive Oil**: Contains healthy fats and antioxidants.

Lifestyle Changes for Immune Support

1. **Regular Exercise**:
    - **Benefits**: Boosts immune function and overall health.
    - **Examples**: Engage in activities such as walking, jogging, or yoga.
2. **Adequate Sleep**:
    - **Purpose**: Supports immune function and helps the body recover from illnesses.
    - **Guideline**: Aim for 7-9 hours of quality sleep each night and maintain a consistent sleep schedule.
3. **Stress Management**:
    - **Importance**: Reduces the impact of stress on the immune system.
    - **Techniques**: Practice relaxation techniques such as mindfulness, deep breathing, and meditation.
4. **Good Hygiene Practices**:
    - **Purpose**: Reduces the risk of infections and supports overall health.
    - **Guideline**: Practice regular handwashing, avoid touching the face, and avoid sharing personal items.
5. **Hydration**:
    - **Importance**: Maintains overall health and supports the body's recovery from infections.
    - **Guideline**: Drink plenty of water throughout the day and consider herbal teas for additional benefits.

6. **Avoid Smoking and Limit Alcohol**:
   - **Reason**: Smoking and excessive alcohol consumption can weaken the immune system.
   - **Guideline**: Avoid smoking and limit alcohol intake to support immune health.

Additional Therapies

1. **Acupuncture**:
   - **Benefits**: May help with symptom management, boost immune function, and support overall well-being.

2. **Massage Therapy**:
   - **Usage**: Can help alleviate symptoms, improve circulation, and support overall health.

3. **Biofeedback**:
   - **Purpose**: Helps manage stress and physiological responses.

4. **Reiki or Energy Healing**:
   - **Benefits**: Supports relaxation and overall well-being.

5. **Naturopathic Medicine**:
   - **Purpose**: Offers a holistic approach to managing symptoms and supporting overall health.

Conclusion

Supporting the immune system and managing symptoms of flu and viral infections holistically involves a multi-faceted approach that includes dietary adjustments, herbal remedies, lifestyle changes, and supportive therapies. By incorporating these strategies, you can enhance immune function, support recovery, and improve overall health. Always consult with a healthcare provider before starting any new treatment plan or making significant changes to your current regimen.

Bacterial Infections

Bacterial infections occur when harmful bacteria invade the body, leading to various symptoms and health issues. Holistic management of bacterial infections involves a combination of dietary adjustments, herbal remedies, lifestyle changes, and supportive therapies to support the body's natural defenses and aid in recovery.

Key Herbs for Bacterial Infections

1. **Garlic (Allium sativum)**:
   - **Properties**: Antimicrobial, antibacterial.
   - **Usage**: Consumed raw, added to food, or taken as a supplement to help combat bacterial infections and support immune health.

2. **Echinacea (Echinacea purpurea)**:
   - **Properties**: Immune-boosting, antibacterial.
   - **Usage**: Taken as a supplement or in tea to support the immune system and help manage bacterial infections.

3. **Goldenseal (Hydrastis canadensis)**:
   - **Properties**: Antibacterial, antimicrobial.
   - **Usage**: Consumed as a supplement or in tea to help fight bacterial infections and support overall health.

4. **Oregano Oil (Origanum vulgare)**:
   - **Properties**: Antibacterial, antiviral.
   - **Usage**: Taken as a supplement or diluted in water for topical application to help manage bacterial infections.

5. **Ginger (Zingiber officinale)**:
   - **Properties**: Antibacterial, anti-inflammatory.
   - **Usage**: Used in tea or added to foods to support immune health and help alleviate symptoms of bacterial infections.

6. **Cranberry (Vaccinium macrocarpon)**:
   - **Properties**: Antibacterial, supports urinary tract health.
   - **Usage**: Consumed as juice or in supplement form to help prevent and manage urinary tract infections (UTIs) caused by bacteria.

Dietary Recommendations for Supporting Recovery from Bacterial Infections

1. **Antioxidant-Rich Foods**:
   - **Purpose**: Supports immune function and helps combat oxidative stress.
   - **Include**:
     - **Berries**: Blueberries, strawberries, and raspberries.
     - **Nuts and Seeds**: Almonds, walnuts, and chia seeds.

- **Vegetables**: Spinach, kale, and bell peppers.

2. **Probiotic Foods**:
   - **Importance**: Supports gut health and helps restore beneficial bacteria after antibiotic use.
   - **Include**:
     - **Yogurt**: Contains live cultures beneficial for gut health.
     - **Kefir**: Fermented dairy with probiotics.
     - **Fermented Vegetables**: Sauerkraut, kimchi, and pickles.

3. **Hydrating Foods and Fluids**:
   - **Purpose**: Maintains hydration and supports overall health.
   - **Include**:
     - **Soups and Broths**: Provide hydration and nutrients.
     - **Watermelon**: High water content and vitamins.
     - **Herbal Teas**: Support hydration and provide additional health benefits.

4. **Lean Proteins**:
   - **Importance**: Supports immune function and tissue repair.
   - **Include**:
     - **Chicken**: Lean protein source.
     - **Tofu**: Plant-based protein.
     - **Legumes**: Beans, lentils, and chickpeas.

5. **Whole Grains**:
   - **Purpose**: Provides sustained energy and supports digestive health.
   - **Include**:
     - **Quinoa**: High in protein and nutrients.
     - **Brown Rice**: Provides fiber and essential minerals.
     - **Oats**: Supports heart health and digestion.

6. **Anti-Inflammatory Foods**:
   - **Importance**: Reduces inflammation and supports immune health.

- Include:
  - **Turmeric**: Contains curcumin, which has anti-inflammatory properties.
  - **Green Tea**: Rich in antioxidants and anti-inflammatory compounds.
  - **Olive Oil**: Contains healthy fats and antioxidants.

Lifestyle Changes for Supporting Recovery

1. **Regular Exercise**:
   - **Benefits**: Supports immune function and overall health.
   - **Examples**: Engage in activities such as walking, jogging, or yoga.

2. **Adequate Sleep**:
   - **Purpose**: Supports immune function and helps the body recover from infections.
   - **Guideline**: Aim for 7-9 hours of quality sleep each night and maintain a consistent sleep schedule.

3. **Stress Management**:
   - **Importance**: Reduces the impact of stress on the immune system.
   - **Techniques**: Practice relaxation techniques such as mindfulness, deep breathing, and meditation.

4. **Good Hygiene Practices**:
   - **Purpose**: Reduces the risk of infections and supports overall health.
   - **Guideline**: Practice regular handwashing, avoid touching the face, and avoid sharing personal items.

5. **Hydration**:
   - **Importance**: Maintains overall health and supports the body's recovery from infections.
   - **Guideline**: Drink plenty of water throughout the day and consider herbal teas for additional benefits.

6. **Avoid Smoking and Limit Alcohol**:
   - **Reason**: Smoking and excessive alcohol consumption can weaken the immune system.

- **Guideline**: Avoid smoking and limit alcohol intake to support immune health.

Additional Therapies

1. **Acupuncture**:
   - **Benefits**: May help with symptom management, boost immune function, and support overall well-being.

2. **Massage Therapy**:
   - **Usage**: Can help alleviate symptoms, improve circulation, and support overall health.

3. **Biofeedback**:
   - **Purpose**: Helps manage stress and physiological responses.

4. **Reiki or Energy Healing**:
   - **Benefits**: Supports relaxation and overall well-being.

5. **Naturopathic Medicine**:
   - **Purpose**: Offers a holistic approach to managing bacterial infections and supporting overall health.

Conclusion

Managing bacterial infections holistically involves a multi-faceted approach that includes dietary adjustments, herbal remedies, lifestyle changes, and supportive therapies. By incorporating these strategies, you can support your body's natural defenses, aid in recovery, and improve overall health. Always consult with a healthcare provider before starting any new treatment plan or making significant changes to your current regimen.

Psoriasis and Eczema

Psoriasis and eczema are chronic skin conditions characterized by inflammation, itching, and skin changes. Managing these conditions holistically involves a combination of dietary adjustments, herbal remedies, lifestyle changes, and supportive therapies to reduce inflammation, support skin health, and alleviate symptoms.

Key Herbs for Psoriasis and Eczema

1. **Aloe Vera (Aloe barbadensis)**:
   - **Properties**: Soothing, anti-inflammatory.

- **Usage**: Applied topically as a gel to soothe irritated skin and reduce inflammation.

2. **Turmeric (Curcuma longa)**:
   - **Properties**: Anti-inflammatory, antioxidant.
   - **Usage**: Consumed as a supplement or in food to help reduce inflammation and support skin health.

3. **Calendula (Calendula officinalis)**:
   - **Properties**: Anti-inflammatory, skin-healing.
   - **Usage**: Used topically as an ointment or cream to help soothe and heal irritated skin.

4. **Chamomile (Matricaria chamomilla)**:
   - **Properties**: Anti-inflammatory, soothing.
   - **Usage**: Applied topically as a compress or used in bath soaks to help calm irritated skin.

5. **Evening Primrose Oil (Oenothera biennis)**:
   - **Properties**: Anti-inflammatory, skin-nourishing.
   - **Usage**: Taken as a supplement or applied topically to help manage symptoms and improve skin condition.

6. **Witch Hazel (Hamamelis virginiana)**:
   - **Properties**: Astringent, anti-inflammatory.
   - **Usage**: Applied topically to help reduce itching and inflammation.

Dietary Recommendations for Psoriasis and Eczema

1. **Anti-Inflammatory Foods**:
   - **Purpose**: Reduces inflammation and supports skin health.
   - **Include**:
     - **Fatty Fish**: Salmon, mackerel, and sardines.
     - **Nuts and Seeds**: Walnuts, chia seeds, and flaxseeds.
     - **Fruits and Vegetables**: Berries, leafy greens, and bell peppers.

2. **Omega-3 Fatty Acids**:
   - **Importance**: Supports skin health and reduces inflammation.

- Include:
  - **Flaxseeds**: Ground or as oil.
  - **Chia Seeds**: Added to smoothies or oatmeal.
  - **Fish Oil**: Supplements or through fatty fish.

3. **Vitamin D-Rich Foods**:
   - **Purpose**: Supports skin health and immune function.
   - Include:
     - **Fatty Fish**: Salmon, mackerel, and sardines.
     - **Fortified Foods**: Fortified milk, orange juice, and cereals.
     - **Eggs**: Provide vitamin D and other essential nutrients.

4. **Probiotic Foods**:
   - **Importance**: Supports gut health, which can influence skin conditions.
   - Include:
     - **Yogurt**: Contains live cultures beneficial for gut health.
     - **Kefir**: Fermented dairy with probiotics.
     - **Fermented Vegetables**: Sauerkraut, kimchi, and pickles.

5. **Hydrating Foods**:
   - **Purpose**: Maintains skin hydration and supports overall health.
   - Include:
     - **Cucumbers**: Hydrating and low in calories.
     - **Watermelon**: High water content and vitamins.
     - **Leafy Greens**: Provides hydration and essential nutrients.

6. **Avoid Trigger Foods**:
   - **Importance**: Identifying and avoiding foods that may trigger flare-ups.
   - **Examples**: Common triggers can include dairy, gluten, or processed foods.

Lifestyle Changes for Managing Psoriasis and Eczema

1. **Regular Moisturization**:
   - **Benefits**: Helps maintain skin hydration and prevent dryness.

- **Recommendation**: Use emollients or moisturizers daily to keep skin hydrated.

2. **Avoid Irritants**:
    - **Purpose**: Reduces skin irritation and flare-ups.
    - **Guideline**: Avoid harsh soaps, detergents, and chemicals. Opt for gentle, fragrance-free products.

3. **Stress Management**:
    - **Importance**: Reduces the impact of stress on skin conditions.
    - **Techniques**: Practice relaxation techniques such as mindfulness, deep breathing, and meditation.

4. **Avoid Hot Water**:
    - **Reason**: Hot water can strip the skin of natural oils and worsen symptoms.
    - **Guideline**: Use lukewarm water for bathing and showering.

5. **Wear Soft, Breathable Fabrics**:
    - **Purpose**: Reduces skin irritation and promotes comfort.
    - **Recommendation**: Choose fabrics like cotton and avoid wool or synthetic materials that can irritate the skin.

6. **Adequate Hydration**:
    - **Importance**: Maintains skin hydration and supports overall health.
    - **Guideline**: Drink plenty of water throughout the day.

Additional Therapies

1. **Phototherapy**:
    - **Benefits**: Can help manage psoriasis and eczema by exposing the skin to controlled amounts of ultraviolet light.

2. **Acupuncture**:
    - **Usage**: May help with symptom management and support overall skin health.

3. **Massage Therapy**:
    - **Benefits**: Can help alleviate stress and improve circulation, potentially benefiting skin health.

4. **Biofeedback**:
   - **Purpose**: Helps manage stress and physiological responses related to skin conditions.

5. **Reiki or Energy Healing**:
   - **Benefits**: Supports relaxation and overall well-being.

6. **Naturopathic Medicine**:
   - **Purpose**: Offers a holistic approach to managing symptoms and supporting skin health.

Conclusion

Managing psoriasis and eczema holistically involves a multi-faceted approach that includes dietary adjustments, herbal remedies, lifestyle changes, and supportive therapies. By incorporating these strategies, you can help reduce inflammation, support skin health, and alleviate symptoms. Always consult with a healthcare provider before starting any new treatment plan or making significant changes to your current regimen.

Vertigo and Tinnitus

Vertigo and tinnitus are conditions that affect the inner ear and auditory system. Vertigo involves a sensation of spinning or dizziness, while tinnitus is characterized by ringing or other sounds in the ears. Holistic management of these conditions involves a combination of dietary adjustments, herbal remedies, lifestyle changes, and supportive therapies to alleviate symptoms and support overall health.

Key Herbs for Vertigo and Tinnitus

1. **Gingko Biloba (Gingko biloba)**:
   - **Properties**: Improves circulation, antioxidant.
   - **Usage**: Taken as a supplement to support blood flow to the brain and ears, which may help with symptoms of vertigo and tinnitus.

2. **Ginger (Zingiber officinale)**:
   - **Properties**: Anti-inflammatory, improves circulation.
   - **Usage**: Consumed as tea or added to foods to help alleviate dizziness and nausea associated with vertigo.

3. **Cayenne Pepper (Capsicum annuum)**:
   - **Properties**: Improves circulation, reduces inflammation.

- **Usage**: Added to foods or taken in supplement form to support blood flow and reduce symptoms of vertigo.

4. **Hawthorn (Crataegus spp.)**:
   - **Properties**: Supports cardiovascular health, improves circulation.
   - **Usage**: Taken as a supplement or in tea to support overall circulation, which may benefit those with vertigo.

5. **Black Cohosh (Actaea racemosa)**:
   - **Properties**: May help with dizziness and ear-related symptoms.
   - **Usage**: Taken as a supplement under the guidance of a healthcare provider.

6. **Peppermint (Mentha piperita)**:
   - **Properties**: Soothing, anti-inflammatory.
   - **Usage**: Used in tea or as an essential oil for its calming effects on the digestive system, which may help with symptoms of vertigo.

Dietary Recommendations for Supporting Vertigo and Tinnitus

1. **Hydrating Foods and Fluids**:
   - **Purpose**: Maintains hydration and supports overall health.
   - **Include**:
     - **Water**: Drink plenty of water throughout the day.
     - **Cucumbers**: High water content.
     - **Watermelon**: Hydrating and high in vitamins.

2. **Low-Sodium Diet**:
   - **Importance**: Helps manage fluid balance in the body and may alleviate symptoms of vertigo.
   - **Include**:
     - **Fruits and Vegetables**: Fresh and unprocessed.
     - **Lean Proteins**: Chicken, fish, and legumes.
     - **Whole Grains**: Brown rice, quinoa, and oats.

3. **Avoid Caffeine and Alcohol**:
   - **Reason**: Caffeine and alcohol can exacerbate symptoms of vertigo and tinnitus.

- **Guideline**: Limit or avoid consumption of caffeinated beverages and alcohol.

4. **Anti-Inflammatory Foods**:
    - **Purpose**: Reduces inflammation and supports overall health.
    - **Include**:
        - **Fatty Fish**: Salmon, mackerel, and sardines.
        - **Nuts and Seeds**: Walnuts, chia seeds, and flaxseeds.
        - **Leafy Greens**: Spinach, kale, and Swiss chard.

5. **Vitamin and Mineral-Rich Foods**:
    - **Importance**: Supports overall health and may help manage symptoms.
    - **Include**:
        - **Vitamin B12**: Found in lean meats, dairy products, and fortified cereals.
        - **Magnesium**: Found in nuts, seeds, and leafy greens.
        - **Vitamin C**: Found in citrus fruits, berries, and bell peppers.

6. **Ginger and Turmeric**:
    - **Purpose**: Reduces inflammation and supports circulation.
    - **Include**:
        - **Ginger**: Used in teas or added to foods.
        - **Turmeric**: Used in cooking or as a supplement.

Lifestyle Changes for Managing Vertigo and Tinnitus

1. **Balance Exercises**:
    - **Benefits**: Helps improve coordination and reduce dizziness.
    - **Examples**: Engage in activities such as Tai Chi, balance training, or specific vestibular exercises.

2. **Stress Management**:
    - **Importance**: Reduces the impact of stress on symptoms.
    - **Techniques**: Practice relaxation techniques such as mindfulness, deep breathing, and meditation.

3. **Adequate Sleep**:

- **Purpose**: Supports overall health and helps manage symptoms.
- **Guideline**: Aim for 7-9 hours of quality sleep each night and maintain a consistent sleep schedule.

4. **Avoid Triggers**:
   - **Reason**: Identifying and avoiding triggers that may worsen symptoms.
   - **Examples**: Avoid sudden movements, loud noises, or positions that exacerbate vertigo.

5. **Healthy Hydration**:
   - **Importance**: Maintains fluid balance and supports overall health.
   - **Guideline**: Drink plenty of water throughout the day.

6. **Hearing Protection**:
   - **Purpose**: Protects ears from loud noises that can aggravate tinnitus.
   - **Guideline**: Use earplugs or noise-cancelling headphones in noisy environments.

Additional Therapies

1. **Vestibular Rehabilitation Therapy (VRT)**:
   - **Benefits**: A type of physical therapy designed to help manage vertigo and improve balance.

2. **Cognitive Behavioral Therapy (CBT)**:
   - **Purpose**: Helps manage the psychological impact of chronic tinnitus and vertigo.

3. **Acupuncture**:
   - **Benefits**: May help alleviate symptoms of vertigo and tinnitus by promoting balance and relaxation.

4. **Sound Therapy**:
   - **Usage**: Helps manage tinnitus by providing background noise or white noise to mask ringing or buzzing sounds.

5. **Biofeedback**:
   - **Purpose**: Helps manage stress and physiological responses related to vertigo and tinnitus.

6. **Reiki or Energy Healing**:

- **Benefits**: Supports relaxation and overall well-being.

Conclusion

Managing vertigo and tinnitus holistically involves a comprehensive approach that includes dietary adjustments, herbal remedies, lifestyle changes, and supportive therapies. By incorporating these strategies, you can help alleviate symptoms, support overall health, and improve quality of life. Always consult with a healthcare provider before starting any new treatment plan or making significant changes to your current regimen.

Thyroid Health

The thyroid is a butterfly-shaped gland located at the base of the neck that plays a crucial role in regulating metabolism, energy levels, and overall hormonal balance. Thyroid health is vital for maintaining overall well-being, and managing thyroid conditions holistically involves a combination of dietary adjustments, herbal remedies, lifestyle changes, and supportive therapies to support thyroid function and overall health.

Key Herbs for Thyroid Health

1. **Ashwagandha (Withania somnifera)**:
   - **Properties**: Adaptogen, supports thyroid function.
   - **Usage**: Taken as a supplement to help balance thyroid hormones and reduce stress.

2. **Bladderwrack (Fucus vesiculosus)**:
   - **Properties**: Rich in iodine, supports thyroid health.
   - **Usage**: Taken as a supplement or in powdered form to provide iodine, which is essential for thyroid function.

3. **Guggul (Commiphora wightii)**:
   - **Properties**: Supports thyroid function, reduces inflammation.
   - **Usage**: Taken as a supplement to help regulate thyroid hormones and support overall thyroid health.

4. **Coleus Forskohlii (Coleus barbatus)**:
   - **Properties**: Supports thyroid function, boosts metabolism.
   - **Usage**: Taken as a supplement to support thyroid health and metabolic function.

5. **Nettle Leaf (Urtica dioica)**:

- **Properties**: Supports overall thyroid health, anti-inflammatory.
- **Usage**: Consumed as tea or in supplement form to support thyroid function and reduce inflammation.

6. **Licorice Root (Glycyrrhiza glabra)**:
   - **Properties**: Balances cortisol levels, supports adrenal and thyroid health.
   - **Usage**: Taken as a supplement or in tea to support hormonal balance and overall thyroid function.

Dietary Recommendations for Supporting Thyroid Health

1. **Iodine-Rich Foods**:
   - **Importance**: Iodine is essential for thyroid hormone production.
   - **Include**:
     - **Sea Vegetables**: Seaweed, such as kelp and nori.
     - **Iodized Salt**: Use iodized salt in cooking.
     - **Fish**: Salmon, cod, and tuna.

2. **Selenium-Rich Foods**:
   - **Purpose**: Supports thyroid function and hormone metabolism.
   - **Include**:
     - **Brazil Nuts**: High in selenium.
     - **Sunflower Seeds**: Provide selenium and other nutrients.
     - **Eggs**: Contain selenium and other essential nutrients.

3. **Zinc-Rich Foods**:
   - **Importance**: Supports thyroid hormone production and immune function.
   - **Include**:
     - **Pumpkin Seeds**: Rich in zinc.
     - **Shellfish**: Oysters and crab.
     - **Legumes**: Chickpeas and lentils.

4. **Anti-Inflammatory Foods**:
   - **Purpose**: Reduces inflammation and supports overall health.
   - **Include**:

- **Fatty Fish**: Salmon, mackerel, and sardines.
- **Leafy Greens**: Spinach, kale, and Swiss chard.
- **Berries**: Blueberries, strawberries, and raspberries.

5. **Whole Foods and Balanced Diet**:
   - **Importance**: Supports overall health and thyroid function.
   - **Include**:
     - **Lean Proteins**: Chicken, fish, and legumes.
     - **Whole Grains**: Brown rice, quinoa, and oats.
     - **Fresh Fruits and Vegetables**: Provides essential vitamins and minerals.

6. **Avoid Goitrogens in Excess**:
   - **Reason**: Goitrogens can interfere with iodine absorption and thyroid function.
   - **Examples**: Common goitrogenic foods include raw cruciferous vegetables like broccoli, cabbage, and Brussels sprouts. Cooking these vegetables can reduce their goitrogenic effects.

Lifestyle Changes for Supporting Thyroid Health

1. **Regular Exercise**:
   - **Benefits**: Supports metabolism and overall thyroid health.
   - **Examples**: Engage in activities such as walking, jogging, strength training, or yoga.

2. **Stress Management**:
   - **Importance**: Reduces the impact of stress on thyroid function and overall health.
   - **Techniques**: Practice relaxation techniques such as mindfulness, deep breathing, and meditation.

3. **Adequate Sleep**:
   - **Purpose**: Supports hormonal balance and overall health.
   - **Guideline**: Aim for 7-9 hours of quality sleep each night and maintain a consistent sleep schedule.

4. **Avoid Environmental Toxins**:

- **Reason**: Toxins can impact thyroid health and function.
- **Guideline**: Reduce exposure to chemicals and pollutants, and opt for natural or organic products when possible.

5. **Maintain a Healthy Weight**:
   - **Importance**: Supports metabolic function and overall health.
   - **Guideline**: Achieve and maintain a healthy weight through balanced diet and regular exercise.

6. **Hydration**:
   - **Purpose**: Maintains overall health and supports thyroid function.
   - **Guideline**: Drink plenty of water throughout the day.

Additional Therapies

1. **Thyroid Hormone Replacement Therapy**:
   - **Purpose**: Prescribed by healthcare providers for individuals with thyroid hormone deficiencies.

2. **Acupuncture**:
   - **Benefits**: May help with symptoms related to thyroid dysfunction and support overall well-being.

3. **Naturopathic Medicine**:
   - **Purpose**: Offers a holistic approach to supporting thyroid health and managing thyroid conditions.

4. **Biofeedback**:
   - **Usage**: Helps manage stress and physiological responses related to thyroid health.

5. **Reiki or Energy Healing**:
   - **Benefits**: Supports relaxation and overall well-being.

Conclusion

Supporting thyroid health holistically involves a multi-faceted approach that includes dietary adjustments, herbal remedies, lifestyle changes, and supportive therapies. By incorporating these strategies, you can help maintain optimal thyroid function, support overall health, and improve quality of life. Always consult with a healthcare provider before starting any new treatment plan or making significant changes to your current regimen.

Allergies

Allergies occur when the immune system overreacts to normally harmless substances, known as allergens, resulting in symptoms such as sneezing, itching, congestion, and more severe reactions. Holistic management of allergies involves a combination of dietary adjustments, herbal remedies, lifestyle changes, and supportive therapies to help reduce symptoms and improve overall well-being.

Key Herbs for Allergies

1. **Stinging Nettle (Urtica dioica)**:
    - **Properties**: Antihistamine, anti-inflammatory.
    - **Usage**: Taken as a supplement or in tea to help alleviate allergy symptoms and reduce inflammation.

2. **Butterbur (Petasites hybridus)**:
    - **Properties**: Antihistamine, reduces nasal congestion.
    - **Usage**: Taken as a supplement to help manage symptoms of seasonal allergies and reduce inflammation.

3. **Quercetin (from fruits and vegetables such as apples and onions)**:
    - **Properties**: Natural antihistamine, anti-inflammatory.
    - **Usage**: Consumed through dietary sources or as a supplement to help reduce histamine release and manage allergy symptoms.

4. **Elderflower (Sambucus nigra)**:
    - **Properties**: Anti-inflammatory, immune-supporting.
    - **Usage**: Used in tea or as a tincture to support the immune system and reduce allergy symptoms.

5. **Chamomile (Matricaria chamomilla)**:
    - **Properties**: Anti-inflammatory, soothing.
    - **Usage**: Used in tea or applied topically to alleviate symptoms such as itching and irritation.

6. **Licorice Root (Glycyrrhiza glabra)**:
    - **Properties**: Anti-inflammatory, supports adrenal function.
    - **Usage**: Taken as a supplement or in tea to help balance the immune system and reduce inflammation.

Dietary Recommendations for Managing Allergies

1. **Anti-Inflammatory Foods**:
   - **Purpose**: Reduces overall inflammation and supports immune health.
   - **Include**:
     - **Fatty Fish**: Salmon, mackerel, and sardines.
     - **Leafy Greens**: Spinach, kale, and Swiss chard.
     - **Berries**: Blueberries, strawberries, and raspberries.

2. **Vitamin C-Rich Foods**:
   - **Importance**: Supports the immune system and acts as a natural antihistamine.
   - **Include**:
     - **Citrus Fruits**: Oranges, grapefruits, and lemons.
     - **Bell Peppers**: High in vitamin C and antioxidants.
     - **Kiwi**: Rich in vitamin C and other nutrients.

3. **Omega-3 Fatty Acids**:
   - **Purpose**: Reduces inflammation and supports immune health.
   - **Include**:
     - **Flaxseeds**: Ground or as oil.
     - **Chia Seeds**: Added to smoothies or oatmeal.
     - **Walnuts**: Provide omega-3s and other nutrients.

4. **Probiotic Foods**:
   - **Importance**: Supports gut health and can influence the immune system.
   - **Include**:
     - **Yogurt**: Contains live cultures beneficial for gut health.
     - **Kefir**: Fermented dairy with probiotics.
     - **Fermented Vegetables**: Sauerkraut, kimchi, and pickles.

5. **Hydrating Foods**:
   - **Purpose**: Helps maintain hydration and support overall health.

- Include:
    - **Cucumbers**: High water content.
    - **Watermelon**: Hydrating and high in vitamins.
    - **Celery**: Provides hydration and essential nutrients.

6. **Avoid Common Allergens**:
    - **Reason**: Identifying and avoiding foods that may trigger allergic reactions.
    - **Examples**: Common allergens include dairy, gluten, nuts, and shellfish.

Lifestyle Changes for Managing Allergies

1. **Allergen Avoidance**:
    - **Purpose**: Reduces exposure to triggers that can worsen symptoms.
    - **Guideline**: Identify and avoid common allergens such as pollen, dust mites, and pet dander.

2. **Regular Cleaning**:
    - **Benefits**: Reduces allergen exposure in the home.
    - **Examples**: Regularly clean carpets, bedding, and other areas where allergens may accumulate.

3. **Air Purification**:
    - **Purpose**: Reduces allergens in indoor air.
    - **Guideline**: Use air purifiers with HEPA filters to help remove airborne allergens.

4. **Humidity Control**:
    - **Importance**: Helps reduce mold and dust mites, which can trigger allergies.
    - **Guideline**: Maintain indoor humidity levels between 30-50% and use a dehumidifier if needed.

5. **Nasal Irrigation**:
    - **Purpose**: Cleanses nasal passages and reduces allergy symptoms.
    - **Guideline**: Use a saline nasal rinse or neti pot to help clear allergens from the nasal passages.

6. **Regular Exercise**:
    - **Benefits**: Supports overall health and may help reduce allergy symptoms.

- **Examples**: Engage in outdoor activities when pollen counts are low, and consider indoor exercises if outdoor allergens are high.

Additional Therapies

1. **Acupuncture**:
   - **Benefits**: May help alleviate allergy symptoms by balancing the immune system and reducing inflammation.

2. **Allergy Testing and Immunotherapy**:
   - **Purpose**: Identifies specific allergens and provides targeted treatment through desensitization.

3. **Biofeedback**:
   - **Usage**: Helps manage stress and physiological responses related to allergies.

4. **Reiki or Energy Healing**:
   - **Benefits**: Supports relaxation and overall well-being, which may help manage allergy symptoms.

5. **Naturopathic Medicine**:
   - **Purpose**: Offers a holistic approach to managing allergies and supporting overall health.

Conclusion

Managing allergies holistically involves a comprehensive approach that includes dietary adjustments, herbal remedies, lifestyle changes, and supportive therapies. By incorporating these strategies, you can help reduce symptoms, support immune health, and improve quality of life. Always consult with a healthcare provider before starting any new treatment plan or making significant changes to your current regimen.

Alzheimer's and Dementia

Alzheimer's disease and dementia are progressive neurological conditions that affect memory, cognition, and overall brain function. Holistic management of Alzheimer's and dementia involves a multi-faceted approach, including dietary adjustments, herbal remedies, lifestyle changes, and supportive therapies to support brain health and improve quality of life.

Key Herbs for Alzheimer's and Dementia

1. **Ginkgo Biloba (Ginkgo biloba)**:
   - **Properties**: Improves circulation, cognitive function.

- **Usage**: Taken as a supplement to enhance blood flow to the brain and support cognitive function.

2. **Turmeric (Curcuma longa)**:
    - **Properties**: Anti-inflammatory, antioxidant.
    - **Usage**: Consumed as a spice in food or taken in supplement form to support brain health and reduce inflammation.

3. **Bacopa (Bacopa monnieri)**:
    - **Properties**: Cognitive enhancer, reduces anxiety.
    - **Usage**: Taken as a supplement to improve memory and cognitive function.

4. **Rosemary (Rosmarinus officinalis)**:
    - **Properties**: Cognitive support, antioxidant.
    - **Usage**: Used in cooking or as an essential oil to support memory and overall brain health.

5. **Ashwagandha (Withania somnifera)**:
    - **Properties**: Adaptogen, supports stress reduction.
    - **Usage**: Taken as a supplement to help manage stress and support cognitive function.

6. **Sage (Salvia officinalis)**:
    - **Properties**: Cognitive support, antioxidant.
    - **Usage**: Used in cooking or as a supplement to support brain health and memory.

Dietary Recommendations for Supporting Brain Health

1. **Omega-3 Fatty Acids**:
    - **Importance**: Supports brain function and cognitive health.
    - **Include**:
        - **Fatty Fish**: Salmon, mackerel, and sardines.
        - **Flaxseeds**: Ground or as oil.
        - **Chia Seeds**: Added to smoothies or oatmeal.

2. **Antioxidant-Rich Foods**:
    - **Purpose**: Protects brain cells from oxidative stress and inflammation.

- Include:
    - **Berries**: Blueberries, strawberries, and raspberries.
    - **Dark Chocolate**: Contains antioxidants and may support cognitive function.
    - **Nuts**: Walnuts and almonds.
3. **Whole Grains**:
    - **Importance**: Provides essential nutrients and supports overall brain health.
    - Include:
        - **Oats**: For breakfast or snacks.
        - **Quinoa**: As a side dish or salad base.
        - **Brown Rice**: Adds fiber and nutrients to meals.
4. **Leafy Greens**:
    - **Purpose**: Rich in vitamins and minerals that support brain health.
    - Include:
        - **Spinach**: Adds to salads, smoothies, or as a side dish.
        - **Kale**: Used in salads, soups, or smoothies.
        - **Swiss Chard**: Added to soups or sautéed as a side.
5. **Healthy Fats**:
    - **Importance**: Supports brain function and overall health.
    - Include:
        - **Avocados**: Used in salads, sandwiches, or as a spread.
        - **Olive Oil**: Used in cooking or as a salad dressing.
        - **Nuts and Seeds**: Added to meals or snacks.
6. **Hydrating Foods**:
    - **Purpose**: Supports overall health and cognitive function.
    - Include:
        - **Cucumbers**: High water content.
        - **Watermelon**: Hydrating and high in vitamins.

- **Celery**: Provides hydration and essential nutrients.

Lifestyle Changes for Supporting Brain Health

1. **Regular Physical Exercise**:
   - **Benefits**: Supports brain health, improves cognitive function, and enhances overall well-being.
   - **Examples**: Engage in activities such as walking, swimming, or strength training.

2. **Mental Stimulation**:
   - **Importance**: Keeps the brain active and engaged.
   - **Examples**: Engage in puzzles, reading, learning new skills, or playing cognitive games.

3. **Social Engagement**:
   - **Purpose**: Supports emotional well-being and cognitive function.
   - **Examples**: Participate in social activities, join clubs, or volunteer in the community.

4. **Stress Management**:
   - **Importance**: Reduces the impact of stress on brain health.
   - **Techniques**: Practice relaxation techniques such as mindfulness, meditation, or yoga.

5. **Adequate Sleep**:
   - **Purpose**: Supports cognitive function and overall brain health.
   - **Guideline**: Aim for 7-9 hours of quality sleep each night and maintain a consistent sleep schedule.

6. **Healthy Hydration**:
   - **Importance**: Supports overall health and cognitive function.
   - **Guideline**: Drink plenty of water throughout the day.

Additional Therapies

1. **Cognitive Behavioral Therapy (CBT)**:
   - **Purpose**: Helps manage symptoms related to cognitive decline and supports emotional well-being.

2. **Acupuncture**:
   - **Benefits**: May help support cognitive function and overall brain health.
3. **Music Therapy**:
   - **Purpose**: Enhances emotional well-being and cognitive function through music.
4. **Art Therapy**:
   - **Benefits**: Supports cognitive and emotional health through creative expression.
5. **Naturopathic Medicine**:
   - **Purpose**: Offers a holistic approach to supporting brain health and managing symptoms of Alzheimer's and dementia.

Conclusion

Supporting brain health and managing Alzheimer's and dementia holistically involves a comprehensive approach that includes dietary adjustments, herbal remedies, lifestyle changes, and supportive therapies. By incorporating these strategies, you can help maintain cognitive function, support overall well-being, and improve quality of life. Always consult with a healthcare provider before starting any new treatment plan or making significant changes to your current regimen.

Heart Health

Maintaining heart health is crucial for overall well-being and longevity. Holistic management of heart health involves a combination of dietary adjustments, herbal remedies, lifestyle changes, and supportive therapies to support cardiovascular function and reduce the risk of heart disease.

Key Herbs for Heart Health

1. **Hawthorn (Crataegus monogyna)**:
   - **Properties**: Supports cardiovascular health, improves circulation.
   - **Usage**: Taken as a supplement or in tea to help strengthen the heart and improve blood flow.
2. **Garlic (Allium sativum)**:
   - **Properties**: Reduces cholesterol, supports blood pressure regulation.
   - **Usage**: Consumed raw, cooked, or in supplement form to support cardiovascular health.

3. **Ginger (Zingiber officinale)**:
   - **Properties**: Reduces inflammation, supports circulation.
   - **Usage**: Used in cooking or as a tea to help support heart health and reduce inflammation.

4. **Turmeric (Curcuma longa)**:
   - **Properties**: Anti-inflammatory, antioxidant.
   - **Usage**: Consumed as a spice in food or taken in supplement form to support heart health and reduce inflammation.

5. **Green Tea (Camellia sinensis)**:
   - **Properties**: Antioxidant, supports healthy blood pressure and cholesterol levels.
   - **Usage**: Consumed as tea to support cardiovascular health and reduce oxidative stress.

6. **Cinnamon (Cinnamomum verum)**:
   - **Properties**: Supports healthy blood sugar levels, reduces inflammation.
   - **Usage**: Used in cooking or as a supplement to help manage blood sugar levels and support heart health.

Dietary Recommendations for Supporting Heart Health

1. **Omega-3 Fatty Acids**:
   - **Importance**: Supports heart health by reducing inflammation and improving lipid profiles.
   - **Include**:
     - **Fatty Fish**: Salmon, mackerel, and sardines.
     - **Flaxseeds**: Ground or as oil.
     - **Chia Seeds**: Added to smoothies or oatmeal.

2. **Whole Grains**:
   - **Purpose**: Supports heart health by providing fiber and essential nutrients.
   - **Include**:
     - **Oats**: For breakfast or snacks.
     - **Quinoa**: As a side dish or salad base.

- **Brown Rice**: Adds fiber and nutrients to meals.
3. **Fruits and Vegetables**:
    - **Importance**: Rich in vitamins, minerals, and antioxidants that support heart health.
    - **Include**:
        - **Berries**: Blueberries, strawberries, and raspberries.
        - **Leafy Greens**: Spinach, kale, and Swiss chard.
        - **Citrus Fruits**: Oranges, grapefruits, and lemons.
4. **Nuts and Seeds**:
    - **Purpose**: Provide healthy fats, fiber, and nutrients that support heart health.
    - **Include**:
        - **Walnuts**: High in omega-3 fatty acids.
        - **Almonds**: Provide healthy fats and fiber.
        - **Pumpkin Seeds**: Rich in magnesium and other nutrients.
5. **Legumes**:
    - **Importance**: Support heart health by providing fiber and plant-based protein.
    - **Include**:
        - **Chickpeas**: Used in salads, stews, or hummus.
        - **Lentils**: Added to soups, stews, or as a side dish.
        - **Black Beans**: Used in salads, soups, or as a side dish.
6. **Healthy Fats**:
    - **Purpose**: Supports cardiovascular health and overall well-being.
    - **Include**:
        - **Avocados**: Used in salads, sandwiches, or as a spread.
        - **Olive Oil**: Used in cooking or as a salad dressing.
        - **Nuts and Seeds**: Added to meals or snacks.

Lifestyle Changes for Supporting Heart Health

1. **Regular Physical Exercise**:

- **Benefits**: Supports cardiovascular health, helps manage weight, and reduces risk factors for heart disease.
- **Examples**: Engage in activities such as walking, jogging, swimming, or strength training.

2. **Stress Management**:
   - **Importance**: Reduces the impact of stress on cardiovascular health.
   - **Techniques**: Practice relaxation techniques such as mindfulness, meditation, or yoga.

3. **Healthy Weight Management**:
   - **Purpose**: Supports overall cardiovascular health and reduces the risk of heart disease.
   - **Guideline**: Maintain a healthy weight through balanced diet and regular exercise.

4. **Adequate Sleep**:
   - **Importance**: Supports overall health and cardiovascular function.
   - **Guideline**: Aim for 7-9 hours of quality sleep each night and maintain a consistent sleep schedule.

5. **Avoid Smoking and Limit Alcohol Consumption**:
   - **Reason**: Reduces risk factors for heart disease and supports overall health.
   - **Guideline**: Avoid smoking and limit alcohol consumption to moderate levels.

6. **Regular Health Screenings**:
   - **Purpose**: Monitors cardiovascular health and identifies risk factors early.
   - **Guideline**: Schedule regular check-ups with your healthcare provider to monitor blood pressure, cholesterol levels, and other cardiovascular health indicators.

Additional Therapies

1. **Acupuncture**:
   - **Benefits**: May help support cardiovascular health and reduce stress.

2. **Massage Therapy**:
   - **Purpose**: Reduces stress and improves circulation.

3. **Biofeedback**:

- **Usage**: Helps manage stress and physiological responses related to heart health.

4. **Naturopathic Medicine**:
    - **Purpose**: Offers a holistic approach to supporting cardiovascular health and managing risk factors for heart disease.

5. **Mind-Body Techniques**:
    - **Benefits**: Supports emotional well-being and overall cardiovascular health.
    - **Examples**: Practice techniques such as guided imagery, progressive muscle relaxation, or tai chi.

Conclusion

Supporting heart health holistically involves a comprehensive approach that includes dietary adjustments, herbal remedies, lifestyle changes, and supportive therapies. By incorporating these strategies, you can help maintain cardiovascular function, support overall well-being, and reduce the risk of heart disease. Always consult with a healthcare provider before starting any new treatment plan or making significant changes to your current regimen.

Menopause Support

Menopause marks the end of a woman's reproductive years and is characterized by the cessation of menstrual cycles and a decline in hormone levels. Managing menopause holistically involves addressing physical, emotional, and lifestyle changes to alleviate symptoms and support overall well-being.

Key Herbs for Menopause Support

1. **Black Cohosh (Cimicifuga racemosa)**:
    - **Properties**: Supports hormonal balance, reduces hot flashes.
    - **Usage**: Taken as a supplement to help manage hot flashes and other menopausal symptoms.

2. **Red Clover (Trifolium pratense)**:
    - **Properties**: Contains phytoestrogens, supports hormonal balance.
    - **Usage**: Consumed as a tea or in supplement form to help alleviate symptoms like hot flashes and mood swings.

3. **Dong Quai (Angelica sinensis)**:
    - **Properties**: Supports hormonal balance, reduces menstrual discomfort.

- **Usage**: Taken as a supplement to help with symptoms related to menopause and support overall hormonal health.

4. **Evening Primrose Oil (Oenothera biennis)**:
   - **Properties**: Contains gamma-linolenic acid (GLA), supports hormonal balance.
   - **Usage**: Taken as a supplement to help manage symptoms like hot flashes and mood swings.

5. **Chaste Tree (Vitex agnus-castus)**:
   - **Properties**: Supports hormonal balance, reduces symptoms of PMS and menopause.
   - **Usage**: Taken as a supplement to help regulate menstrual cycles and alleviate menopausal symptoms.

6. **Ginseng (Panax ginseng)**:
   - **Properties**: Supports energy levels, reduces stress.
   - **Usage**: Taken as a supplement to help manage fatigue and improve overall well-being during menopause.

Dietary Recommendations for Menopause Support

1. **Phytoestrogen-Rich Foods**:
   - **Importance**: Helps balance hormones and alleviate symptoms.
   - **Include**:
     - **Soy Products**: Tofu, tempeh, and soy milk.
     - **Flaxseeds**: Ground or as oil.
     - **Sesame Seeds**: Added to salads or meals.

2. **Calcium-Rich Foods**:
   - **Purpose**: Supports bone health, which can be affected by menopause.
   - **Include**:
     - **Leafy Greens**: Kale, spinach, and collard greens.
     - **Dairy Products**: Yogurt, cheese, and milk.
     - **Fortified Plant Milks**: Almond, soy, or oat milk.

3. **Omega-3 Fatty Acids**:

- **Importance**: Supports heart health and reduces inflammation.
- **Include**:
  - **Fatty Fish**: Salmon, mackerel, and sardines.
  - **Flaxseeds**: Ground or as oil.
  - **Chia Seeds**: Added to smoothies or oatmeal.

4. **Whole Grains**:
   - **Purpose**: Provides fiber and nutrients that support overall health.
   - **Include**:
     - **Oats**: For breakfast or snacks.
     - **Quinoa**: As a side dish or salad base.
     - **Brown Rice**: Adds fiber and nutrients to meals.

5. **Fruits and Vegetables**:
   - **Importance**: Rich in vitamins, minerals, and antioxidants that support overall health.
   - **Include**:
     - **Berries**: Blueberries, strawberries, and raspberries.
     - **Leafy Greens**: Spinach, kale, and Swiss chard.
     - **Citrus Fruits**: Oranges, grapefruits, and lemons.

6. **Hydrating Foods**:
   - **Purpose**: Supports hydration and overall health.
   - **Include**:
     - **Cucumbers**: High water content.
     - **Watermelon**: Hydrating and high in vitamins.
     - **Celery**: Provides hydration and essential nutrients.

Lifestyle Changes for Menopause Support

1. **Regular Physical Exercise**:
   - **Benefits**: Supports overall health, reduces stress, and improves mood.
   - **Examples**: Engage in activities such as walking, swimming, yoga, or strength training.

2. **Stress Management**:
    - **Importance**: Reduces the impact of stress on overall health and well-being.
    - **Techniques**: Practice relaxation techniques such as mindfulness, meditation, or deep breathing exercises.

3. **Adequate Sleep**:
    - **Purpose**: Supports overall health and well-being.
    - **Guideline**: Aim for 7-9 hours of quality sleep each night and maintain a consistent sleep schedule.

4. **Healthy Weight Management**:
    - **Importance**: Supports overall health and reduces the risk of weight-related health issues.
    - **Guideline**: Maintain a healthy weight through balanced diet and regular exercise.

5. **Hydration**:
    - **Purpose**: Supports overall health and helps manage symptoms like hot flashes.
    - **Guideline**: Drink plenty of water throughout the day.

6. **Avoid Caffeine and Alcohol**:
    - **Reason**: Can exacerbate symptoms like hot flashes and disrupt sleep.
    - **Guideline**: Limit intake of caffeine and alcohol and opt for healthier alternatives.

Additional Therapies

1. **Acupuncture**:
    - **Benefits**: May help alleviate symptoms like hot flashes, mood swings, and insomnia.

2. **Yoga and Tai Chi**:
    - **Purpose**: Supports physical health, reduces stress, and improves flexibility and balance.

3. **Biofeedback**:
    - **Usage**: Helps manage physiological responses related to menopause symptoms.

4. **Naturopathic Medicine**:
    - **Purpose**: Offers a holistic approach to managing symptoms and supporting overall health during menopause.

5. **Counseling or Support Groups**:
    - **Benefits**: Provides emotional support and helps manage the psychological aspects of menopause.

Conclusion

Supporting heart health holistically involves a comprehensive approach that includes dietary adjustments, herbal remedies, lifestyle changes, and supportive therapies. By incorporating these strategies, you can help maintain cardiovascular function, support overall well-being, and reduce the risk of heart disease. Always consult with a healthcare provider before starting any new treatment plan or making significant changes to your current regimen.

Men's Sexual Health

Men's sexual health encompasses a range of issues including libido, erectile function, fertility, and overall sexual well-being. Holistic management of sexual health involves addressing physical, emotional, and lifestyle factors to support optimal sexual function and overall health.

Key Herbs for Men's Sexual Health

1. **Tribulus Terrestris (Tribulus terrestris)**:
    - **Properties**: Enhances libido, supports testosterone levels.
    - **Usage**: Taken as a supplement to improve sexual desire and support hormonal balance.

2. **Ginseng (Panax ginseng)**:
    - **Properties**: Boosts energy, supports erectile function.
    - **Usage**: Taken as a supplement to improve sexual performance and increase energy levels.

3. **Horny Goat Weed (Epimedium grandiflorum)**:
    - **Properties**: Supports libido, enhances erectile function.
    - **Usage**: Taken as a supplement to improve sexual desire and support overall sexual health.

4. **Maca Root (Lepidium meyenii)**:

- **Properties**: Enhances libido, supports energy levels.
- **Usage**: Consumed as a powder or supplement to boost sexual desire and energy.

5. **Saw Palmetto (Serenoa repens)**:
   - **Properties**: Supports prostate health, reduces symptoms of benign prostatic hyperplasia (BPH).
   - **Usage**: Taken as a supplement to support prostate health and improve sexual function.

6. **L-Arginine**:
   - **Properties**: Supports erectile function, enhances blood flow.
   - **Usage**: Taken as a supplement to improve blood flow and support erectile function.

Dietary Recommendations for Men's Sexual Health

1. **Omega-3 Fatty Acids**:
   - **Importance**: Supports cardiovascular health and improves blood flow.
   - **Include**:
     - **Fatty Fish**: Salmon, mackerel, and sardines.
     - **Flaxseeds**: Ground or as oil.
     - **Chia Seeds**: Added to smoothies or oatmeal.

2. **Zinc-Rich Foods**:
   - **Purpose**: Supports testosterone levels and overall sexual health.
   - **Include**:
     - **Oysters**: High in zinc and support sexual function.
     - **Pumpkin Seeds**: Rich in zinc and other nutrients.
     - **Nuts**: Almonds and cashews.

3. **Antioxidant-Rich Foods**:
   - **Importance**: Reduces oxidative stress and supports overall health.
   - **Include**:
     - **Berries**: Blueberries, strawberries, and raspberries.

- **Dark Chocolate**: Contains antioxidants and supports blood flow.
- **Leafy Greens**: Spinach, kale, and Swiss chard.

4. **Healthy Fats**:
   - **Purpose**: Supports overall health and hormone production.
   - **Include**:
     - **Avocados**: Provides healthy fats and supports hormonal health.
     - **Olive Oil**: Used in cooking or as a salad dressing.
     - **Nuts and Seeds**: Added to meals or snacks.

5. **Lean Proteins**:
   - **Importance**: Supports muscle health and overall energy levels.
   - **Include**:
     - **Chicken**: Lean source of protein.
     - **Turkey**: Provides protein and supports overall health.
     - **Legumes**: Beans and lentils for plant-based protein.

6. **Hydrating Foods**:
   - **Purpose**: Supports overall health and energy levels.
   - **Include**:
     - **Cucumbers**: High water content.
     - **Watermelon**: Hydrating and high in vitamins.
     - **Celery**: Provides hydration and essential nutrients.

Lifestyle Changes for Men's Sexual Health

1. **Regular Physical Exercise**:
   - **Benefits**: Supports cardiovascular health, improves blood flow, and boosts energy levels.
   - **Examples**: Engage in activities such as walking, jogging, swimming, or strength training.

2. **Stress Management**:
   - **Importance**: Reduces the impact of stress on sexual function and overall health.

- **Techniques**: Practice relaxation techniques such as mindfulness, meditation, or deep breathing exercises.

3. **Adequate Sleep**:
   - **Purpose**: Supports overall health and hormone production.
   - **Guideline**: Aim for 7-9 hours of quality sleep each night and maintain a consistent sleep schedule.

4. **Healthy Weight Management**:
   - **Importance**: Supports overall health and reduces the risk of weight-related health issues.
   - **Guideline**: Maintain a healthy weight through balanced diet and regular exercise.

5. **Limit Alcohol and Avoid Smoking**:
   - **Reason**: Excessive alcohol and smoking can impair sexual function and overall health.
   - **Guideline**: Limit alcohol consumption and avoid smoking to support sexual health.

6. **Hydration**:
   - **Purpose**: Supports overall health and maintains energy levels.
   - **Guideline**: Drink plenty of water throughout the day.

Additional Therapies

1. **Counseling or Therapy**:
   - **Benefits**: Helps address psychological and emotional aspects related to sexual health.

2. **Acupuncture**:
   - **Purpose**: May help improve sexual function and reduce stress.

3. **Massage Therapy**:
   - **Benefits**: Reduces stress and improves overall well-being.

4. **Naturopathic Medicine**:
   - **Purpose**: Offers a holistic approach to supporting sexual health and addressing underlying issues.

5. **Sexual Health Education**:

- **Importance**: Provides information and strategies for improving sexual function and overall well-being.

Conclusion

Supporting men's sexual health holistically involves a comprehensive approach that includes dietary adjustments, herbal remedies, lifestyle changes, and supportive therapies. By incorporating these strategies, you can help improve sexual function, support overall health, and enhance quality of life. Always consult with a healthcare provider before starting any new treatment plan or making significant changes to your current regimen.

Sleep Disorders

Sleep disorders affect the quality and quantity of sleep, impacting overall health and well-being. Holistic management of sleep disorders involves addressing underlying causes and incorporating natural strategies to improve sleep quality and promote restful sleep.

Key Herbs for Sleep Disorders

1. **Valerian Root (Valeriana officinalis)**:
   - **Properties**: Promotes relaxation, supports sleep quality.
   - **Usage**: Taken as a supplement or tea to help improve sleep onset and duration.

2. **Chamomile (Matricaria chamomilla)**:
   - **Properties**: Calming, supports relaxation and sleep.
   - **Usage**: Consumed as a tea to help promote restful sleep and reduce anxiety.

3. **Lavender (Lavandula angustifolia)**:
   - **Properties**: Calming, supports relaxation and sleep.
   - **Usage**: Used in aromatherapy or as a tea to help improve sleep quality.

4. **Passionflower (Passiflora incarnata)**:
   - **Properties**: Reduces anxiety, supports relaxation.
   - **Usage**: Taken as a supplement or tea to help manage insomnia and promote relaxation.

5. **Lemon Balm (Melissa officinalis)**:
   - **Properties**: Calming, supports relaxation and sleep.
   - **Usage**: Consumed as a tea or supplement to help reduce sleep disturbances.

6. **California Poppy (Eschscholzia californica)**:
   - **Properties**: Supports relaxation, reduces anxiety.
   - **Usage**: Taken as a supplement to help improve sleep quality and reduce restlessness.

Dietary Recommendations for Better Sleep

1. **Magnesium-Rich Foods**:
   - **Importance**: Supports relaxation and helps with sleep quality.
   - **Include**:
     - **Leafy Greens**: Spinach, kale.
     - **Nuts and Seeds**: Almonds, pumpkin seeds.
     - **Whole Grains**: Brown rice, quinoa.

2. **Tryptophan-Rich Foods**:
   - **Purpose**: Supports serotonin production, which aids sleep.
   - **Include**:
     - **Turkey**: High in tryptophan.
     - **Pumpkin Seeds**: Rich in tryptophan and magnesium.
     - **Bananas**: Contains tryptophan and magnesium.

3. **Complex Carbohydrates**:
   - **Importance**: Helps increase serotonin levels and supports sleep.
   - **Include**:
     - **Oats**: For breakfast or snacks.
     - **Sweet Potatoes**: As a side dish.
     - **Whole Grain Bread**: Added to meals.

4. **Hydrating Foods**:
   - **Purpose**: Supports overall hydration and sleep quality.
   - **Include**:
     - **Cucumbers**: High water content.
     - **Watermelon**: Hydrating and high in vitamins.

- **Celery**: Provides hydration and essential nutrients.

5. **Avoid Caffeine and Heavy Meals Before Bed**:
   - **Reason**: Caffeine and heavy meals can disrupt sleep.
   - **Guideline**: Avoid consuming caffeine and large meals in the hours leading up to bedtime.

Lifestyle Changes for Better Sleep

1. **Establish a Consistent Sleep Schedule**:
   - **Benefits**: Helps regulate your internal clock and improve sleep quality.
   - **Guideline**: Go to bed and wake up at the same time every day, even on weekends.

2. **Create a Relaxing Bedtime Routine**:
   - **Purpose**: Signals to your body that it's time to wind down.
   - **Techniques**: Incorporate activities such as reading, taking a warm bath, or practicing relaxation techniques.

3. **Optimize Your Sleep Environment**:
   - **Importance**: A comfortable and conducive environment supports better sleep.
   - **Tips**:
     - **Comfortable Bedding**: Ensure your mattress and pillows are supportive and comfortable.
     - **Dark and Cool Room**: Use blackout curtains and keep the room cool.
     - **Limit Noise**: Use earplugs or white noise machines if needed.

4. **Limit Exposure to Screens Before Bed**:
   - **Reason**: Blue light from screens can interfere with sleep.
   - **Guideline**: Avoid using electronic devices such as phones, tablets, and computers at least an hour before bed.

5. **Physical Activity**:
   - **Benefits**: Regular exercise supports better sleep quality.
   - **Examples**: Engage in activities such as walking, swimming, or yoga, but avoid vigorous exercise close to bedtime.

6. **Manage Stress and Anxiety**:
    - **Importance**: Reduces the impact of stress on sleep.
    - **Techniques**: Practice mindfulness, meditation, or deep breathing exercises to help manage stress levels.

Additional Therapies

1. **Cognitive Behavioral Therapy for Insomnia (CBT-I)**:
    - **Benefits**: Helps address thoughts and behaviors that affect sleep.
2. **Aromatherapy**:
    - **Purpose**: Uses essential oils like lavender to promote relaxation and improve sleep quality.
3. **Acupuncture**:
    - **Benefits**: May help improve sleep quality and reduce insomnia.
4. **Massage Therapy**:
    - **Purpose**: Reduces stress and promotes relaxation.
5. **Naturopathic Medicine**:
    - **Purpose**: Offers a holistic approach to managing sleep disorders and improving sleep quality.

Conclusion

Managing sleep disorders holistically involves a comprehensive approach that includes dietary adjustments, herbal remedies, lifestyle changes, and supportive therapies. By incorporating these strategies, you can improve sleep quality, address underlying issues, and support overall health and well-being. Always consult with a healthcare provider before starting any new treatment plan or making significant changes to your current regimen.

Weight Loss

Achieving and maintaining a healthy weight involves a combination of balanced nutrition, regular physical activity, and lifestyle changes. A holistic approach to weight loss focuses on addressing the root causes of weight gain, supporting metabolic health, and promoting sustainable habits.

Key Herbs for Weight Loss

1. **Green Tea (Camellia sinensis)**:

- **Properties**: Boosts metabolism, supports fat oxidation.
- **Usage**: Consumed as tea or in supplement form to enhance fat burning and support weight loss.

2. **Garcinia Cambogia (Garcinia cambogia)**:
   - **Properties**: Suppresses appetite, inhibits fat production.
   - **Usage**: Taken as a supplement to reduce appetite and support weight management.

3. **Cinnamon (Cinnamomum verum)**:
   - **Properties**: Regulates blood sugar levels, supports metabolism.
   - **Usage**: Added to meals or beverages to help manage blood sugar and reduce cravings.

4. **Ginger (Zingiber officinale)**:
   - **Properties**: Supports digestion, boosts metabolism.
   - **Usage**: Consumed as tea or added to meals to aid digestion and enhance metabolism.

5. **Dandelion (Taraxacum officinale)**:
   - **Properties**: Supports detoxification, promotes digestion.
   - **Usage**: Taken as tea or in supplement form to support liver function and aid weight loss.

6. **Fennel (Foeniculum vulgare)**:
   - **Properties**: Reduces bloating, supports digestion.
   - **Usage**: Consumed as tea or in supplement form to help reduce bloating and support digestive health.

Dietary Recommendations for Weight Loss

1. **High-Fiber Foods**:
   - **Importance**: Supports satiety and reduces overall calorie intake.
   - **Include**:
     - **Vegetables**: Leafy greens, broccoli, and carrots.
     - **Fruits**: Apples, berries, and pears.
     - **Whole Grains**: Oats, quinoa, and brown rice.

2. **Lean Proteins**:
   - **Purpose**: Supports muscle health and aids in satiety.
   - **Include**:
     - **Chicken Breast**: Lean source of protein.
     - **Turkey**: Provides protein and supports overall health.
     - **Legumes**: Beans, lentils, and chickpeas.
3. **Healthy Fats**:
   - **Importance**: Supports overall health and helps manage cravings.
   - **Include**:
     - **Avocados**: Provides healthy fats and supports satiety.
     - **Olive Oil**: Used in cooking or as a salad dressing.
     - **Nuts and Seeds**: Almonds, chia seeds, and flaxseeds.
4. **Hydrating Foods**:
   - **Purpose**: Supports hydration and helps manage appetite.
   - **Include**:
     - **Cucumbers**: High water content.
     - **Watermelon**: Hydrating and low in calories.
     - **Celery**: Provides hydration and essential nutrients.
5. **Balanced Meals**:
   - **Importance**: Supports steady energy levels and prevents overeating.
   - **Guideline**: Include a balance of protein, healthy fats, and complex carbohydrates in each meal.
6. **Limit Processed Foods and Sugars**:
   - **Reason**: Processed foods and sugars can contribute to weight gain and unhealthy eating habits.
   - **Guideline**: Focus on whole, unprocessed foods and reduce intake of sugary snacks and beverages.

Lifestyle Changes for Weight Loss

1. **Regular Physical Activity**:

- **Benefits**: Supports calorie burning, improves metabolism, and enhances overall health.
- **Examples**: Engage in activities such as walking, running, strength training, or group fitness classes.

2. **Portion Control**:
   - **Importance**: Helps manage calorie intake and supports weight loss.
   - **Tips**: Use smaller plates, be mindful of portion sizes, and avoid eating large portions of high-calorie foods.

3. **Mindful Eating**:
   - **Purpose**: Supports healthy eating habits and reduces overeating.
   - **Techniques**: Eat slowly, savor each bite, and listen to your body's hunger and fullness cues.

4. **Adequate Sleep**:
   - **Benefits**: Supports overall health and helps regulate metabolism.
   - **Guideline**: Aim for 7-9 hours of quality sleep each night and maintain a consistent sleep schedule.

5. **Stress Management**:
   - **Importance**: Reduces emotional eating and supports overall well-being.
   - **Techniques**: Practice relaxation techniques such as mindfulness, meditation, or deep breathing exercises.

6. **Hydration**:
   - **Purpose**: Supports metabolism and helps manage appetite.
   - **Guideline**: Drink plenty of water throughout the day and limit intake of sugary beverages.

Additional Therapies

1. **Behavioral Therapy**:
   - **Benefits**: Helps address eating habits, emotional eating, and supports sustainable weight loss.

2. **Acupuncture**:
   - **Purpose**: May help with appetite regulation and support weight management.

3. **Naturopathic Medicine**:
    - **Purpose**: Offers a holistic approach to weight loss, including dietary and lifestyle recommendations.

4. **Nutrition Counseling**:
    - **Benefits**: Provides personalized guidance on healthy eating and weight management strategies.

5. **Support Groups**:
    - **Purpose**: Provides emotional support and motivation through shared experiences and goals.

Conclusion

Achieving and maintaining a healthy weight involves a multifaceted approach that includes dietary adjustments, physical activity, lifestyle changes, and supportive therapies. By incorporating these strategies, you can support weight loss, enhance overall health, and develop sustainable habits for long-term success. Always consult with a healthcare provider before starting any new treatment plan or making significant changes to your current regimen.

Creating Your Personalized Wellness Plan

Assessing Your Health Needs

Assessing your health needs is a crucial first step in creating an effective wellness plan. It involves evaluating your current health status, identifying areas for improvement, and setting specific goals based on your unique circumstances. Here's a guide to help you assess your health needs comprehensively:

1. Conduct a Self-Assessment

1. **Review Your Current Health Status**:
    - **Evaluate**: Your overall health, including any existing medical conditions, symptoms, or concerns.
    - **Consider**: Factors such as weight, blood pressure, blood sugar levels, and cholesterol.

2. **Track Symptoms and Health Issues**:
    - **Record**: Any persistent symptoms or issues (e.g., fatigue, digestive problems, chronic pain).
    - **Note**: When these symptoms occur and any potential triggers.

3. **Assess Lifestyle Factors**:
    - **Review**: Your daily routines, including diet, physical activity, sleep patterns, and stress levels.
    - **Identify**: Areas that may be contributing to health issues or where improvements can be made.

2. Set Specific Health Goals

1. **Define Your Objectives**:
    - **Identify**: Clear, specific health goals (e.g., losing weight, improving sleep quality, managing stress).
    - **Make Goals SMART**: Specific, Measurable, Achievable, Relevant, and Time-bound.

2. **Prioritize Your Goals**:
    - **Rank**: Your goals based on importance and urgency.
    - **Focus**: On achieving one or two goals at a time to ensure progress.

3. Consult with Healthcare Professionals

1. **Schedule a Check-Up:**
   - **Visit**: Your primary care physician or a specialist for a comprehensive health evaluation.
   - **Discuss**: Any symptoms, concerns, or goals you have.

2. **Get Diagnostic Tests:**
   - **Request**: Tests or screenings as recommended by your healthcare provider to assess your health status (e.g., blood tests, imaging).

3. **Seek Expert Advice:**
   - **Consult**: With nutritionists, fitness trainers, or other specialists for personalized recommendations.

4. Evaluate Your Mental and Emotional Health

1. **Assess Stress Levels:**
   - **Identify**: Sources of stress and how they impact your well-being.
   - **Evaluate**: Stress management strategies and their effectiveness.

2. **Consider Emotional Well-being:**
   - **Reflect**: On your mood, emotional health, and any symptoms of anxiety or depression.
   - **Seek Support**: If needed, consider therapy or counseling services.

3. **Review Social Connections:**
   - **Examine**: Your relationships and social support network.
   - **Consider**: How social interactions impact your health and well-being.

5. Review and Adjust Lifestyle Factors

1. **Diet and Nutrition:**
   - **Evaluate**: Your current eating habits and nutritional intake.
   - **Identify**: Areas for improvement, such as incorporating more whole foods or reducing processed foods.

2. **Physical Activity:**
   - **Assess**: Your current exercise routine and physical activity levels.
   - **Set Goals**: For increasing activity or incorporating different types of exercise.

3. **Sleep and Rest**:
    - **Review**: Your sleep patterns and quality.
    - **Identify**: Factors that may be affecting your sleep and consider improvements.
4. **Hydration**:
    - **Evaluate**: Your daily water intake and hydration levels.
    - **Ensure**: You are drinking enough water and minimizing dehydrating beverages.

6. Create a Health Action Plan

1. **Develop a Plan**:
    - **Include**: Specific actions, resources, and timelines to achieve your health goals.
    - **Incorporate**: Recommendations from healthcare professionals and lifestyle changes.
2. **Set Milestones**:
    - **Define**: Key milestones and checkpoints to track your progress.
    - **Monitor**: Your achievements and make adjustments as needed.
3. **Seek Support**:
    - **Engage**: With support groups, wellness coaches, or accountability partners to stay motivated.

7. Regularly Review and Update Your Assessment

1. **Monitor Progress**:
    - **Track**: Changes in symptoms, health metrics, and progress toward goals.
    - **Adjust**: Your plan based on what is working and any new needs or goals.
2. **Update Your Plan**:
    - **Revise**: Your health action plan as needed to reflect changes in your health status or goals.
    - **Consult**: With healthcare professionals periodically to ensure your plan remains effective.

Conclusion

Assessing your health needs involves a comprehensive evaluation of your current health status, setting specific goals, consulting with healthcare professionals, and reviewing lifestyle factors. By following these steps, you can develop a personalized wellness plan that addresses your unique needs and supports your overall well-being. Regular monitoring and adjustments will help you stay on track and achieve your health goals.

Choosing the Right Protocols

Selecting the appropriate protocols for your wellness plan involves identifying effective strategies and practices that address your specific health needs and goals. Here's a guide to help you choose the right protocols for your personalized wellness plan:

1. Identify Your Health Goals and Needs

1. **Define Your Objectives**:
   - **Clarify**: Your primary health goals (e.g., managing chronic pain, improving digestive health, supporting mental well-being).
   - **Prioritize**: The most pressing needs or conditions you want to address.
2. **Assess Health Conditions**:
   - **Review**: Any existing health conditions or symptoms you are experiencing.
   - **Consult**: With healthcare professionals to understand your specific needs and potential protocols.

2. Research and Evaluate Protocols

1. **Understand Protocol Options**:
   - **Research**: Different types of protocols available for your health goals (e.g., herbal remedies, dietary changes, exercise routines).
   - **Evaluate**: The effectiveness, safety, and evidence supporting each protocol.
2. **Consider Holistic Approaches**:
   - **Explore**: Comprehensive approaches that integrate multiple strategies (e.g., combining nutrition, exercise, and stress management).
   - **Assess**: How these approaches align with your overall wellness plan.

3. Tailor Protocols to Your Needs

1. **Personalize Protocols**:
   - **Customize**: Protocols to fit your individual preferences, lifestyle, and health status.

- **Adjust**: Based on any allergies, intolerances, or contraindications.

2. **Start with Small Changes**:
    - **Implement**: A few protocols at a time to assess their impact and effectiveness.
    - **Monitor**: Your response to each protocol and make adjustments as needed.

4. Integrate Protocols into Your Wellness Plan

1. **Create a Routine**:
    - **Schedule**: The chosen protocols into your daily or weekly routine.
    - **Set Reminders**: To ensure consistency in following the protocols.
2. **Combine Protocols Effectively**:
    - **Integrate**: Different protocols in a way that complements and supports each other (e.g., combining herbal remedies with dietary changes).
    - **Avoid Conflicts**: Ensure that the protocols do not counteract each other or cause adverse interactions.

5. Monitor and Adjust Your Protocols

1. **Track Progress**:
    - **Record**: Any changes in symptoms, health metrics, and overall well-being.
    - **Use**: Journals or apps to keep track of your experiences with each protocol.
2. **Evaluate Effectiveness**:
    - **Assess**: How well the protocols are working towards achieving your health goals.
    - **Seek Feedback**: From healthcare professionals or wellness coaches.
3. **Make Adjustments**:
    - **Revise**: Protocols based on your progress and any new needs or goals.
    - **Consult**: With professionals if you need guidance on modifying your protocols.

6. Consider Lifestyle and Practicality

1. **Assess Feasibility**:
    - **Consider**: How practical and manageable each protocol is within your lifestyle.

- **Evaluate**: Time commitments, costs, and ease of implementation.
   2. **Ensure Sustainability**:
      - **Choose**: Protocols that you can realistically maintain over the long term.
      - **Adapt**: Protocols to fit your evolving needs and circumstances.

7. Seek Professional Guidance

1. **Consult with Experts**:
   - **Get Advice**: From healthcare providers, herbalists, nutritionists, or wellness coaches to ensure you are choosing appropriate protocols.
   - **Discuss**: Any concerns or questions about integrating protocols into your plan.
2. **Review Protocols Periodically**:
   - **Schedule Check-Ins**: With professionals to review your progress and make necessary adjustments to your protocols.

Conclusion

Choosing the right protocols involves a thorough understanding of your health needs, researching available options, personalizing and integrating protocols into your wellness plan, and monitoring their effectiveness. By carefully selecting and implementing protocols that align with your goals and lifestyle, you can create a comprehensive and effective wellness plan that supports your overall health and well-being. Regular evaluation and professional guidance will help ensure that your chosen protocols continue to meet your needs and contribute to your success.

Tracking Your Progress

Tracking your progress is essential for evaluating the effectiveness of your wellness plan, staying motivated, and making necessary adjustments. Here's a guide to help you effectively track your progress and achieve your health goals:

1. Set Clear Benchmarks and Goals

1. **Define Specific Goals**:
   - **Specify**: Clear and measurable objectives (e.g., reducing blood pressure, losing 10 pounds, improving sleep quality).
   - **Establish**: Short-term and long-term goals to guide your progress.
2. **Create Milestones**:

- **Identify**: Key milestones that signify progress towards your goals (e.g., achieving a certain number of exercise sessions, reaching a target weight).
- **Set Deadlines**: For achieving these milestones to maintain motivation and focus.

2. Use Tools and Methods for Tracking

1. **Maintain a Health Journal**:
   - **Record**: Daily or weekly entries about your diet, exercise, symptoms, and overall well-being.
   - **Include**: Notes on any changes in mood, energy levels, and specific challenges.

2. **Utilize Apps and Technology**:
   - **Track**: Using health and fitness apps for logging exercise, food intake, sleep patterns, and other health metrics.
   - **Monitor**: Progress through dashboards and analytics provided by the apps.

3. **Keep a Progress Log**:
   - **Document**: Key health metrics such as weight, blood pressure, and glucose levels.
   - **Review**: Regularly to assess trends and changes.

4. **Take Photos**:
   - **Capture**: Progress visually (e.g., changes in body composition) to track physical changes over time.
   - **Use**: Before-and-after photos to visualize progress.

3. Regularly Review and Evaluate

1. **Assess Progress Periodically**:
   - **Schedule**: Regular check-ins (e.g., weekly, monthly) to evaluate your progress towards goals and milestones.
   - **Compare**: Current data with your initial benchmarks and goals.

2. **Evaluate Effectiveness**:
   - **Determine**: How well your wellness plan is working (e.g., improvements in health metrics, achievement of goals).
   - **Identify**: Areas where you may need to make changes or adjustments.

4. Adjust Your Plan as Needed

1. **Modify Protocols**:
   - **Make Changes**: To your wellness plan based on progress and feedback (e.g., adjusting exercise routines, changing dietary plans).
   - **Consult**: With healthcare professionals if significant changes are needed.
2. **Adapt Goals**:
   - **Update**: Your goals and milestones as you progress or if your needs change.
   - **Set New Goals**: Based on achievements and evolving health objectives.

5. Celebrate Achievements

1. **Acknowledge Success**:
   - **Recognize**: Your accomplishments and milestones reached.
   - **Reward**: Yourself for progress made (e.g., treating yourself to something enjoyable).
2. **Reflect on Progress**:
   - **Review**: Your journey and the improvements achieved.
   - **Celebrate**: Successes and the positive impact on your health and well-being.

6. Seek Support and Feedback

1. **Engage with Support Networks**:
   - **Share**: Your progress with friends, family, or support groups for encouragement and motivation.
   - **Participate**: In group activities or forums related to your wellness goals.
2. **Consult with Professionals**:
   - **Seek Advice**: From healthcare providers or wellness coaches to review your progress and make informed adjustments.
   - **Discuss**: Any challenges or concerns to get expert guidance.

Conclusion

Tracking your progress is a critical component of achieving your wellness goals and ensuring the effectiveness of your plan. By setting clear goals, using tools and methods for tracking, regularly reviewing and evaluating your progress, and making necessary adjustments, you can stay on track and continue to improve your health and well-being.

Celebrating your achievements and seeking support from networks and professionals will further enhance your motivation and success.

Herbal Remedies and Supplements

Essential Herbs for Wellness

Herbs have been used for centuries to support health and treat various conditions. Incorporating essential herbs into your wellness routine can enhance overall well-being and address specific health concerns. Here's a guide to some key herbs and their benefits:

1. Echinacea

- **Benefits**:
    - **Immune Support**: Boosts the immune system and helps prevent colds and infections.
    - **Anti-inflammatory**: Reduces inflammation and supports respiratory health.
- **Usage**:
    - **Forms**: Tea, tincture, capsules.
    - **Dosage**: Follow label instructions or consult a healthcare provider.

2. Ginger

- **Benefits**:
    - **Digestive Health**: Aids digestion, reduces nausea, and alleviates bloating.
    - **Anti-inflammatory**: Provides relief from inflammation and pain.
- **Usage**:
    - **Forms**: Fresh root, tea, capsules, dried powder.
    - **Dosage**: Use as needed in cooking or follow supplement guidelines.

3. Turmeric

- **Benefits**:
    - **Anti-inflammatory**: Contains curcumin, which helps reduce inflammation and pain.
    - **Antioxidant**: Protects cells from oxidative stress and supports overall health.
- **Usage**:
    - **Forms**: Fresh root, powder, capsules.

- **Dosage**: Include in cooking or take as a supplement following dosage instructions.

4. Lavender

- **Benefits**:
    - **Relaxation**: Promotes relaxation and improves sleep quality.
    - **Anxiety Reduction**: Helps alleviate symptoms of anxiety and stress.
- **Usage**:
    - **Forms**: Essential oil (for aromatherapy), tea, dried flowers.
    - **Dosage**: Use essential oil in diffusers, tea as needed, or dried flowers for relaxation.

5. Peppermint

- **Benefits**:
    - **Digestive Health**: Eases digestive issues such as bloating and gas.
    - **Pain Relief**: Provides relief from headaches and muscle pain.
- **Usage**:
    - **Forms**: Tea, essential oil, capsules.
    - **Dosage**: Drink tea as needed or use essential oil topically with carrier oil.

6. Chamomile

- **Benefits**:
    - **Sleep Aid**: Promotes restful sleep and relaxation.
    - **Digestive Health**: Soothes digestive issues and reduces bloating.
- **Usage**:
    - **Forms**: Tea, capsules, tincture.
    - **Dosage**: Drink tea before bedtime or follow supplement guidelines.

7. Garlic

- **Benefits**:
    - **Heart Health**: Supports cardiovascular health and helps lower blood pressure.

- o **Immune Support**: Boosts immune function and has antimicrobial properties.
- **Usage**:
  - o **Forms**: Fresh cloves, garlic powder, capsules.
  - o **Dosage**: Incorporate into meals or take supplements following dosage recommendations.

8. Ginseng

- **Benefits**:
  - o **Energy and Vitality**: Enhances energy levels and combats fatigue.
  - o **Cognitive Function**: Supports mental clarity and cognitive function.
- **Usage**:
  - o **Forms**: Root, tea, capsules.
  - o **Dosage**: Follow label instructions or consult a healthcare provider for appropriate dosage.

9. St. John's Wort

- **Benefits**:
  - o **Mood Support**: Helps manage symptoms of mild to moderate depression and anxiety.
  - o **Nerve Health**: Supports nerve health and reduces nerve pain.
- **Usage**:
  - o **Forms**: Capsules, tincture, tea.
  - o **Dosage**: Follow dosage instructions and consult a healthcare provider, especially if taking other medications.

10. Ashwagandha

- **Benefits**:
  - o **Stress Reduction**: Helps manage stress and reduce anxiety.
  - o **Energy and Stamina**: Enhances overall energy levels and stamina.
- **Usage**:
  - o **Forms**: Powder, capsules, tincture.
  - o **Dosage**: Follow supplement guidelines or consult with a healthcare provider.

11. Holy Basil (Tulsi)

- **Benefits**:
  - **Stress Relief**: Supports stress management and overall resilience.
  - **Immune Support**: Enhances immune function and provides antioxidant protection.
- **Usage**:
  - **Forms**: Tea, capsules, fresh leaves.
  - **Dosage**: Drink tea or take supplements following dosage recommendations.

Conclusion

Incorporating essential herbs into your wellness routine can support various aspects of health, from digestive function to stress management. Understanding the benefits and appropriate usage of each herb helps you choose the right ones for your needs. Always consult with a healthcare provider before starting new herbs or supplements, especially if you have existing health conditions or are taking other medications.

How to Make Herbal Remedies

Creating your own herbal remedies can be a rewarding way to support your health using natural ingredients. Here's a guide on how to make various herbal remedies at home, including teas, tinctures, and oils.

1. Herbal Teas

Ingredients:

- Dried herbs or fresh herbs (e.g., chamomile, peppermint, ginger)

Equipment:

- Teapot or heatproof container
- Strainer or infuser

Steps:

1. **Choose Herbs**: Select herbs based on the benefits you seek (e.g., peppermint for digestion, chamomile for relaxation).
2. **Prepare Herbs**: If using dried herbs, measure about 1-2 teaspoons per cup of water. For fresh herbs, use about 1 tablespoon per cup.
3. **Boil Water**: Heat water to a rolling boil.

4. **Steep Herbs**: Place herbs in a teapot or heatproof container. Pour boiling water over the herbs.
5. **Infuse**: Let the herbs steep for 5-10 minutes, depending on desired strength.
6. **Strain**: Remove the herbs using a strainer or infuser.
7. **Serve**: Enjoy your tea as is or with honey, lemon, or other flavorings.

2. Herbal Tinctures

Ingredients:

- Dried or fresh herbs (e.g., echinacea, valerian root)
- Alcohol (e.g., vodka or brandy) or vinegar (for alcohol-free tinctures)

Equipment:

- Glass jar with a tight-fitting lid
- Cheesecloth or strainer
- Dark glass dropper bottles (for storage)

Steps:

1. **Prepare Herbs**: Chop dried herbs into small pieces or use fresh herbs. Fill a glass jar about halfway with the herbs.
2. **Add Liquid**: Pour alcohol or vinegar over the herbs, covering them completely.
3. **Seal and Shake**: Close the jar tightly and shake it well.
4. **Infuse**: Store in a dark, cool place for 4-6 weeks. Shake the jar daily.
5. **Strain**: After the infusion period, strain the herbs using cheesecloth or a fine strainer.
6. **Bottle**: Transfer the tincture to dark glass dropper bottles for storage. Label with the date and type of herb.

3. Herbal Oils

Ingredients:

- Dried herbs (e.g., lavender, calendula)
- Carrier oil (e.g., olive oil, almond oil)

Equipment:

- Glass jar with a tight-fitting lid

- Cheesecloth or strainer
- Glass dropper bottles (for storage)

Steps:

1. **Prepare Herbs:** Chop dried herbs into small pieces and place them in a clean glass jar.
2. **Add Oil:** Pour carrier oil over the herbs, ensuring they are completely covered.
3. **Seal and Infuse:** Close the jar tightly and place it in a warm, sunny spot. Let it infuse for 2-4 weeks, shaking it gently every day.
4. **Strain:** After infusion, strain the herbs out of the oil using cheesecloth or a fine strainer.
5. **Bottle:** Transfer the infused oil to glass dropper bottles. Label with the date and type of herb.

4. Herbal Salves

Ingredients:

- Herbal-infused oil (see Herbal Oils section)
- Beeswax
- Optional: Essential oils (e.g., lavender, tea tree)

Equipment:

- Double boiler or heatproof bowl
- Stirring utensil
- Small containers for storage

Steps:

1. **Melt Beeswax:** In a double boiler, melt beeswax over low heat.
2. **Combine Oil:** Add the herbal-infused oil to the melted beeswax. Use a ratio of about 1 part beeswax to 4 parts oil, adjusting for desired consistency.
3. **Add Essential Oils** (Optional): Add a few drops of essential oils for added benefits and fragrance.
4. **Stir:** Mix thoroughly and pour into small containers.
5. **Cool:** Allow the salve to cool and solidify before sealing the containers.

5. Herbal Vinegars

Ingredients:
- Fresh herbs (e.g., rosemary, thyme)
- Vinegar (e.g., apple cider vinegar, white vinegar)

Equipment:
- Glass jar with a tight-fitting lid
- Strainer
- Glass bottles for storage

Steps:
1. **Prepare Herbs**: Chop fresh herbs and place them in a clean glass jar.
2. **Add Vinegar**: Pour vinegar over the herbs, making sure they are fully covered.
3. **Seal and Infuse**: Close the jar tightly and store in a cool, dark place for 2-4 weeks. Shake the jar occasionally.
4. **Strain**: After infusion, strain the herbs out of the vinegar using a fine strainer.
5. **Bottle**: Transfer the herbal vinegar to glass bottles and label with the date and type of herb.

Conclusion

Making herbal remedies at home allows you to harness the natural benefits of herbs for various health purposes. By following these simple methods for teas, tinctures, oils, salves, and vinegars, you can create effective and personalized remedies. Always ensure that you use high-quality herbs and consult with a healthcare professional if you have any health conditions or are taking other medications.

Supplement Recommendations

Supplements can play a valuable role in supporting overall health and addressing specific needs. However, it's important to choose supplements based on individual health goals and needs. Here's a guide to commonly recommended supplements and their benefits:

1. Multivitamins

- **Benefits**:
  - **Nutrient Support**: Provides a broad spectrum of essential vitamins and minerals.
  - **Fills Gaps**: Helps cover dietary deficiencies and supports overall health.

- **Recommendations**:
    - Choose a high-quality multivitamin tailored to your age, gender, and specific health needs.
    - Look for a balanced formula with bioavailable nutrients.

2. Vitamin D

- **Benefits**:
    - **Bone Health**: Supports calcium absorption and bone strength.
    - **Immune Function**: Enhances immune system function and helps prevent infections.
- **Recommendations**:
    - **Dosage**: Typically 1,000-2,000 IU per day, but consult with a healthcare provider for personalized dosage.
    - **Sources**: Vitamin D3 is often preferred over D2 for better absorption.

3. Omega-3 Fatty Acids

- **Benefits**:
    - **Heart Health**: Supports cardiovascular health by reducing inflammation and triglyceride levels.
    - **Brain Function**: Promotes cognitive health and supports mental well-being.
- **Recommendations**:
    - **Dosage**: 1,000-3,000 mg of combined EPA and DHA per day.
    - **Sources**: Fish oil supplements or algae-based omega-3s (suitable for vegetarians).

4. Probiotics

- **Benefits**:
    - **Digestive Health**: Supports a healthy balance of gut bacteria and improves digestive function.
    - **Immune Support**: Enhances immune system response and may reduce the frequency of infections.
- **Recommendations**:
    - **Strains**: Look for a blend of Lactobacillus and Bifidobacterium strains.

- **Dosage**: 1-10 billion CFU per day, depending on the specific probiotic strain and health need.

5. Magnesium

- **Benefits**:
    - **Muscle Function**: Supports muscle relaxation and reduces cramping.
    - **Sleep Quality**: Enhances sleep quality and helps manage insomnia.
- **Recommendations**:
    - **Dosage**: 200-400 mg per day.
    - **Forms**: Magnesium citrate or glycinate are generally better absorbed than magnesium oxide.

6. Vitamin C

- **Benefits**:
    - **Immune Support**: Boosts immune function and helps prevent common colds.
    - **Antioxidant Protection**: Protects cells from oxidative damage and supports skin health.
- **Recommendations**:
    - **Dosage**: 500-1,000 mg per day.
    - **Sources**: Choose a buffered form or time-release vitamin C for better tolerance.

7. Calcium

- **Benefits**:
    - **Bone Health**: Supports bone density and prevents osteoporosis.
    - **Muscle Function**: Aids in muscle contraction and nerve function.
- **Recommendations**:
    - **Dosage**: 1,000-1,200 mg per day, depending on age and gender.
    - **Forms**: Calcium citrate is better absorbed and may be easier on the stomach than calcium carbonate.

8. Vitamin B12

- **Benefits**:

- o **Energy Production**: Supports red blood cell formation and energy metabolism.
- o **Nerve Health**: Essential for maintaining healthy nerve cells and neurological function.
- **Recommendations**:
  - o **Dosage**: 500-1,000 mcg per day, especially for vegetarians or those with absorption issues.
  - o **Forms**: Methylcobalamin is a preferred form for better bioavailability.

9. Zinc

- **Benefits**:
  - o **Immune Function**: Supports immune system health and wound healing.
  - o **Cell Growth**: Promotes cell division and enzyme function.
- **Recommendations**:
  - o **Dosage**: 15-30 mg per day.
  - o **Forms**: Zinc picolinate or zinc citrate are well-absorbed forms.

10. Coenzyme Q10 (CoQ10)

- **Benefits**:
  - o **Energy Production**: Supports cellular energy production and mitochondrial function.
  - o **Heart Health**: Benefits cardiovascular health and may help manage high blood pressure.
- **Recommendations**:
  - o **Dosage**: 100-200 mg per day.
  - o **Forms**: Ubiquinol is the active form and is better absorbed than ubiquinone.

11. Turmeric/Curcumin

- **Benefits**:
  - o **Anti-inflammatory**: Reduces inflammation and supports joint health.
  - o **Antioxidant**: Provides protection against oxidative stress.
- **Recommendations**:
  - o **Dosage**: 500-1,000 mg of curcumin per day.

- **Forms**: Look for formulations with black pepper (piperine) for enhanced absorption.

Conclusion

When selecting supplements, it's important to consider your individual health needs and consult with a healthcare provider to ensure they are appropriate for you. High-quality supplements can support various aspects of health, from immune function to heart health, but they should complement a balanced diet and healthy lifestyle. Always follow recommended dosages and be mindful of potential interactions with medications or other supplements.

Nutrition for Optimal Health

Anti-Inflammatory Diet

An anti-inflammatory diet focuses on reducing chronic inflammation in the body, which can help prevent and manage various health conditions, such as heart disease, arthritis, and diabetes. This diet emphasizes foods that have anti-inflammatory properties and limits those that can promote inflammation.

1. Core Principles

a. Emphasize Anti-Inflammatory Foods

- **Fruits and Vegetables**: Rich in antioxidants, vitamins, and minerals that combat inflammation.
  - **Examples**: Berries (blueberries, strawberries), leafy greens (spinach, kale), cruciferous vegetables (broccoli, Brussels sprouts), and tomatoes.
- **Whole Grains**: Provide fiber and nutrients that support overall health.
  - **Examples**: Oats, quinoa, brown rice, and barley.
- **Healthy Fats**: Support cellular health and reduce inflammation.
  - **Examples**: Olive oil, avocados, nuts, and seeds.
- **Lean Proteins**: Source of amino acids without the added inflammatory effects of some meats.
  - **Examples**: Fish (especially fatty fish like salmon and mackerel), poultry, legumes, and tofu.
- **Herbs and Spices**: Contain compounds with anti-inflammatory effects.
  - **Examples**: Turmeric, ginger, garlic, and cinnamon.

b. Limit Pro-Inflammatory Foods

- **Refined Carbohydrates**: Can lead to increased inflammation and poor metabolic health.
  - **Examples**: White bread, pastries, sugary cereals, and processed snacks.
- **Added Sugars**: Contribute to inflammation and various health issues.
  - **Examples**: Soda, candy, and sugary desserts.
- **Trans Fats**: Promote inflammation and are linked to heart disease.

- o **Examples**: Margarine, processed foods, and fried foods.
- **Excessive Saturated Fats**: Can increase inflammation and contribute to chronic diseases.
  - o **Examples**: Fatty cuts of red meat, high-fat dairy products, and certain processed meats.
- **Processed and Red Meats**: Often contain additives and high levels of unhealthy fats.
  - o **Examples**: Bacon, sausages, and hot dogs.

2. Sample Meal Plan

a. Breakfast

- **Oatmeal with Berries and Nuts**: Top whole grain oats with blueberries, chia seeds, and a handful of walnuts.
- **Green Smoothie**: Blend spinach, banana, almond milk, and a tablespoon of flaxseeds.

b. Lunch

- **Quinoa Salad**: Mix cooked quinoa with cherry tomatoes, cucumber, bell peppers, avocado, and a lemon-tahini dressing.
- **Grilled Salmon**: Serve with a side of steamed broccoli and a mixed greens salad.

c. Dinner

- **Chicken Stir-Fry**: Cook lean chicken breast with an assortment of vegetables like bell peppers, snap peas, and carrots. Use a sauce made from ginger, garlic, and a splash of low-sodium soy sauce.
- **Sweet Potato**: Roast a sweet potato with a drizzle of olive oil and a sprinkle of turmeric.

d. Snacks

- **Apple Slices with Almond Butter**: Pair a fresh apple with a tablespoon of almond butter.
- **Carrot Sticks with Hummus**: Enjoy fresh carrot sticks dipped in a homemade or store-bought hummus.

3. Hydration

- **Water**: Aim for at least 8 cups (2 liters) of water daily to support overall health and help flush out toxins.

- **Green Tea**: Contains antioxidants and polyphenols that can help reduce inflammation.

4. Lifestyle Considerations

- **Regular Exercise**: Incorporate moderate physical activity, such as walking, swimming, or cycling, to help manage inflammation and support overall health.
- **Stress Management**: Practice stress-reducing techniques like meditation, deep breathing, or yoga to help lower inflammation levels.
- **Adequate Sleep**: Aim for 7-9 hours of quality sleep per night to support recovery and overall well-being.

Conclusion

Adopting an anti-inflammatory diet can help reduce chronic inflammation and improve overall health. By focusing on whole, nutrient-dense foods and minimizing intake of inflammatory ingredients, you can support your body's natural processes and potentially reduce the risk of various health conditions. Always consider consulting a healthcare provider or nutritionist for personalized dietary advice and adjustments based on your individual needs and health status.

Superfoods for Healing

Superfoods are nutrient-dense foods known for their health benefits, particularly in supporting the body's natural healing processes. These foods are rich in vitamins, minerals, antioxidants, and other bioactive compounds that can help prevent disease, boost immunity, and promote overall wellness. Here's a guide to some of the top superfoods for healing:

1. Berries

- **Types**: Blueberries, strawberries, raspberries, blackberries.
- **Benefits**: Rich in antioxidants like anthocyanins and vitamin C, which help combat oxidative stress and inflammation. They support cardiovascular health and improve cognitive function.
- **Ways to Use**: Add to smoothies, yogurt, or oatmeal; use in salads or as a snack.

2. Leafy Greens

- **Types**: Spinach, kale, Swiss chard, arugula.
- **Benefits**: High in vitamins A, C, K, and folate, as well as minerals like iron and calcium. They support immune function, bone health, and detoxification.
- **Ways to Use**: Incorporate into salads, smoothies, soups, and stir-fries.

3. Turmeric

- **Benefits**: Contains curcumin, a powerful anti-inflammatory and antioxidant compound. It supports joint health, reduces inflammation, and may improve cognitive function.
- **Ways to Use**: Add to curries, soups, teas, or smoothies. Consider using with black pepper to enhance absorption.

4. Ginger

- **Benefits**: Known for its anti-inflammatory and antioxidant properties. It aids digestion, supports immune function, and can help alleviate nausea and motion sickness.
- **Ways to Use**: Use fresh ginger in teas, smoothies, stir-fries, or as a spice in cooking.

5. Garlic

- **Benefits**: Contains allicin, which has antimicrobial, anti-inflammatory, and antioxidant properties. Supports cardiovascular health and immune function.
- **Ways to Use**: Add raw or cooked garlic to a variety of dishes, including soups, sauces, and marinades.

6. Chia Seeds

- **Benefits**: High in omega-3 fatty acids, fiber, and antioxidants. They support heart health, digestive health, and blood sugar regulation.
- **Ways to Use**: Add to smoothies, yogurt, oatmeal, or make chia pudding.

7. Nuts and Seeds

- **Types**: Almonds, walnuts, flaxseeds, pumpkin seeds.
- **Benefits**: Rich in healthy fats, protein, vitamins, and minerals. They support heart health, brain function, and provide anti-inflammatory benefits.
- **Ways to Use**: Snack on them, add to salads, or use in baking.

8. Avocado

- **Benefits**: Packed with healthy monounsaturated fats, fiber, vitamins (including vitamin E), and minerals. Supports heart health, skin health, and nutrient absorption.
- **Ways to Use**: Enjoy as a spread, in salads, smoothies, or as a topping for various dishes.

9. Green Tea

- **Benefits**: Contains antioxidants such as catechins, which have anti-inflammatory and anti-cancer properties. Supports metabolism, cognitive function, and cardiovascular health.
- **Ways to Use**: Drink as tea or use in smoothies and recipes.

10. Sweet Potatoes

- **Benefits**: High in vitamins A and C, fiber, and antioxidants. They support eye health, immune function, and digestive health.
- **Ways to Use**: Roast, bake, mash, or add to soups and stews.

11. Quinoa

- **Benefits**: A complete protein source with all nine essential amino acids. High in fiber, magnesium, and antioxidants. Supports muscle health and overall nutrition.
- **Ways to Use**: Use as a base for salads, side dishes, or as a replacement for rice.

12. Beets

- **Benefits**: Rich in betalains, which have anti-inflammatory and antioxidant properties. Support liver health, improve blood flow, and enhance endurance.
- **Ways to Use**: Roast, steam, or add to salads and smoothies.

13. Mushrooms

- **Types**: Shiitake, maitake, reishi, and lion's mane.
- **Benefits**: Contain beta-glucans and other compounds that support immune function, reduce inflammation, and enhance brain health.
- **Ways to Use**: Include in soups, stir-fries, or as a meat substitute in various dishes.

14. Cacao

- **Benefits**: Rich in flavonoids, which have antioxidant and anti-inflammatory effects. Supports cardiovascular health and mood enhancement.
- **Ways to Use**: Add raw cacao powder to smoothies, oatmeal, or use in baking.

Conclusion

Incorporating superfoods into your diet can enhance your body's natural healing processes and support overall health. These nutrient-dense foods provide a range of benefits, from reducing inflammation to improving immune function. Aim to include a variety of these superfoods in your daily diet to maximize their health benefits and support your journey toward optimal wellness.

Lifestyle and Exercise

Stress Reduction Techniques

Stress is a natural part of life, but managing it effectively is crucial for maintaining overall health and well-being. Incorporating stress reduction techniques into your daily routine can help you manage stress more effectively and improve your quality of life. Here are several effective methods for reducing stress:

1. Mindfulness and Meditation

a. Mindfulness Meditation

- **Benefits**: Increases awareness of the present moment, reduces anxiety, and enhances emotional regulation.
- **How to Practice**: Sit quietly and focus on your breath, paying attention to each inhale and exhale. When your mind wanders, gently bring your focus back to your breath.

b. Guided Meditation

- **Benefits**: Provides structure and support for those new to meditation.
- **How to Practice**: Use guided meditation apps or recordings that lead you through relaxation exercises and visualizations.

c. Body Scan Meditation

- **Benefits**: Helps release physical tension and increase body awareness.
- **How to Practice**: Lie down or sit comfortably, then systematically focus on and relax each part of your body, starting from your toes and moving up to your head.

2. Deep Breathing Exercises

a. Diaphragmatic Breathing

- **Benefits**: Promotes relaxation and reduces the physical symptoms of stress.
- **How to Practice**: Breathe deeply through your nose, allowing your abdomen to rise as you fill your lungs with air. Exhale slowly through your mouth, allowing your abdomen to fall.

b. Box Breathing

- **Benefits**: Helps calm the nervous system and improve focus.

- **How to Practice**: Inhale for a count of 4, hold the breath for 4, exhale for 4, and hold the breath out for 4. Repeat several times.

c. 4-7-8 Breathing

- **Benefits**: Reduces anxiety and promotes relaxation.
- **How to Practice**: Inhale through your nose for a count of 4, hold your breath for a count of 7, and exhale slowly through your mouth for a count of 8. Repeat this cycle 4 times.

3. Physical Activity

a. Exercise

- **Benefits**: Boosts mood, reduces stress hormones, and improves overall well-being.
- **Recommendations**: Engage in at least 30 minutes of moderate exercise, such as walking, jogging, or swimming, most days of the week.

b. Yoga

- **Benefits**: Combines physical movement, breath control, and meditation to reduce stress and improve flexibility.
- **How to Practice**: Join a local class or use online resources to practice yoga poses and breathing exercises.

c. Tai Chi

- **Benefits**: Enhances relaxation, balance, and overall health through slow, flowing movements.
- **How to Practice**: Take a class or follow online tutorials to learn Tai Chi forms and techniques.

4. Relaxation Techniques

a. Progressive Muscle Relaxation (PMR)

- **Benefits**: Reduces muscle tension and promotes overall relaxation.
- **How to Practice**: Tense and then slowly release each muscle group in your body, starting from your toes and working up to your head.

b. Visualization

- **Benefits**: Uses mental imagery to promote relaxation and reduce stress.
- **How to Practice**: Close your eyes and imagine a peaceful scene, such as a beach or forest. Focus on the sights, sounds, and sensations of this calming environment.

c. Aromatherapy

- **Benefits**: Uses essential oils to promote relaxation and reduce stress.
- **How to Practice**: Diffuse essential oils like lavender or chamomile in your home, or use them in a warm bath or massage.

5. Lifestyle Adjustments

a. Time Management

- **Benefits**: Reduces stress by improving organization and productivity.
- **How to Practice**: Create a daily schedule, prioritize tasks, and break large tasks into smaller, manageable steps.

b. Healthy Eating

- **Benefits**: Supports overall health and well-being, which can help manage stress.
- **How to Practice**: Eat a balanced diet rich in fruits, vegetables, whole grains, and lean proteins. Limit caffeine, alcohol, and sugar intake.

c. Social Support

- **Benefits**: Provides emotional support and reduces feelings of isolation.
- **How to Practice**: Connect with friends and family regularly, share your feelings, and seek support when needed.

6. Creative Outlets

a. Hobbies and Interests

- **Benefits**: Provides a positive distraction and promotes relaxation.
- **How to Practice**: Engage in activities you enjoy, such as painting, writing, or playing a musical instrument.

b. Journaling

- **Benefits**: Helps process emotions and clarify thoughts.
- **How to Practice**: Write regularly about your thoughts, feelings, and experiences to gain insight and relieve stress.

Conclusion

Incorporating these stress reduction techniques into your daily routine can help manage stress more effectively and improve overall well-being. Experiment with different methods to find what works best for you, and remember that regular practice can lead to long-term benefits. If stress becomes overwhelming, consider seeking professional help from a counselor or therapist.

Exercise Routines for Different Health Conditions

Exercise can play a crucial role in managing and improving various health conditions. Tailoring exercise routines to specific health issues can help alleviate symptoms, enhance overall well-being, and support recovery. Here's a guide to exercise routines for various health conditions:

1. Chronic Pain Management

a. Low-Impact Cardio

- **Examples**: Walking, swimming, cycling.
- **Benefits**: Improves circulation, reduces stiffness, and boosts mood without putting excessive strain on joints.

b. Gentle Stretching

- **Examples**: Yoga poses such as Child's Pose, Cat-Cow, and Seated Forward Bend.
- **Benefits**: Enhances flexibility, reduces muscle tension, and eases pain.

c. Strength Training

- **Examples**: Light weights, resistance bands, bodyweight exercises.
- **Benefits**: Builds muscle strength to support joints and improve function.

2. Inflammatory Bowel Disease (IBD)

a. Low-Impact Exercise

- **Examples**: Walking, stationary cycling, swimming.
- **Benefits**: Helps maintain fitness without exacerbating symptoms.

b. Core Strengthening

- **Examples**: Pelvic tilts, abdominal bracing, gentle Pilates exercises.
- **Benefits**: Strengthens core muscles to support digestion and reduce abdominal discomfort.

c. Flexibility Exercises

- **Examples**: Gentle yoga stretches, foam rolling.
- **Benefits**: Improves flexibility and reduces muscle tension.

3. Brain and Nerve Health

a. Aerobic Exercise

- **Examples**: Brisk walking, jogging, cycling.
- **Benefits**: Enhances cognitive function, supports brain health, and improves mood.

b. Balance Training

- **Examples**: Tai Chi, balance exercises on a stability ball.
- **Benefits**: Improves coordination and reduces the risk of falls.

c. Brain Exercises

- **Examples**: Puzzles, memory games, coordination drills.
- **Benefits**: Stimulates brain activity and cognitive function.

4. Gastroesophageal Reflux Disease (GERD) and Acid Reflux

a. Low-Intensity Cardio

- **Examples**: Walking, low-impact aerobic exercises.
- **Benefits**: Avoids triggering reflux symptoms and supports overall health.

b. Core Strengthening

- **Examples**: Modified planks, leg raises.
- **Benefits**: Strengthens the core without putting pressure on the stomach.

c. Avoiding Exercise Immediately After Meals

- **Recommendations**: Wait at least 1-2 hours after eating before engaging in exercise.

5. Prostate Health

a. Aerobic Exercise

- **Examples**: Walking, jogging, swimming.
- **Benefits**: Supports overall health and can improve urinary function.

b. Pelvic Floor Exercises

- **Examples**: Kegel exercises.
- **Benefits**: Strengthens pelvic muscles and improves urinary control.

c. Gentle Stretching

- **Examples**: Hip stretches, lower back stretches.

- **Benefits**: Reduces muscle tension and supports pelvic health.

6. Lung Health and Chronic Obstructive Pulmonary Disease (COPD)

a. Breathing Exercises

- **Examples**: Diaphragmatic breathing, pursed-lip breathing.
- **Benefits**: Improves lung function and oxygen intake.

b. Low-Intensity Cardio

- **Examples**: Walking, stationary cycling.
- **Benefits**: Enhances cardiovascular health and stamina without overexerting the lungs.

c. Strength Training

- **Examples**: Light weights, resistance bands.
- **Benefits**: Builds muscle strength to support daily activities.

7. Parkinson's Disease

a. Balance and Coordination Exercises

- **Examples**: Tai Chi, balance drills.
- **Benefits**: Improves stability and reduces the risk of falls.

b. Aerobic Exercise

- **Examples**: Walking, swimming, cycling.
- **Benefits**: Supports overall fitness and can improve motor function.

c. Flexibility and Stretching

- **Examples**: Gentle yoga, stretching routines.
- **Benefits**: Maintains flexibility and reduces muscle stiffness.

8. Type-2 Diabetes

a. Cardiovascular Exercise

- **Examples**: Walking, running, swimming.
- **Benefits**: Helps regulate blood sugar levels and improves insulin sensitivity.

b. Strength Training

- **Examples**: Weight lifting, resistance bands.

- **Benefits**: Increases muscle mass, which helps improve glucose metabolism.

c. Flexibility and Stretching

- **Examples**: Yoga, dynamic stretching.
- **Benefits**: Enhances flexibility and reduces muscle tension.

9. Leaky Gut, Gastritis, and Irritable Bowel Syndrome (IBS)

a. Low-Impact Exercise

- **Examples**: Walking, gentle cycling, swimming.
- **Benefits**: Supports digestion and reduces symptoms without causing discomfort.

b. Core Strengthening

- **Examples**: Pelvic tilts, gentle Pilates.
- **Benefits**: Supports abdominal muscles and aids digestion.

c. Stress-Reducing Activities

- **Examples**: Yoga, meditation.
- **Benefits**: Helps manage stress, which can exacerbate digestive issues.

10. Lupus

a. Low-Impact Cardio

- **Examples**: Walking, swimming, stationary cycling.
- **Benefits**: Enhances cardiovascular health and reduces joint stress.

b. Gentle Strength Training

- **Examples**: Light weights, resistance bands.
- **Benefits**: Builds muscle strength without overstraining the body.

c. Flexibility and Stretching

- **Examples**: Yoga, stretching exercises.
- **Benefits**: Maintains joint flexibility and reduces stiffness.

11. Lyme Disease

a. Low-Intensity Cardio

- **Examples**: Walking, gentle cycling.
- **Benefits**: Supports cardiovascular health without exacerbating fatigue.

b. Gentle Stretching

- **Examples**: Light yoga, stretching routines.
- **Benefits**: Reduces muscle stiffness and improves flexibility.

c. Strength Training

- **Examples**: Light resistance exercises.
- **Benefits**: Builds strength and supports overall physical function.

12. Multiple Sclerosis

a. Low-Impact Aerobic Exercise

- **Examples**: Swimming, walking, stationary cycling.
- **Benefits**: Enhances cardiovascular health and reduces fatigue.

b. Balance and Coordination Exercises

- **Examples**: Tai Chi, balance drills.
- **Benefits**: Improves stability and reduces the risk of falls.

c. Flexibility and Stretching

- **Examples**: Gentle yoga, stretching routines.
- **Benefits**: Reduces muscle stiffness and improves range of motion.

13. Adrenal Fatigue

a. Low-Intensity Cardio

- **Examples**: Walking, gentle cycling.
- **Benefits**: Supports overall fitness without overstressing the adrenal glands.

b. Gentle Strength Training

- **Examples**: Bodyweight exercises, light weights.
- **Benefits**: Builds muscle strength and supports energy levels.

c. Relaxation Techniques

- **Examples**: Yoga, meditation.
- **Benefits**: Reduces stress and supports adrenal health.

Conclusion

Tailoring exercise routines to specific health conditions can help manage symptoms, improve overall health, and enhance quality of life. Always consult with a healthcare provider before starting a new exercise regimen, especially if you have a medical condition. Adjust exercise intensity and type based on individual needs and capabilities to ensure safety and effectiveness.

The Importance of Sleep

Sleep is a fundamental component of overall health and well-being. It plays a crucial role in physical, mental, and emotional health, influencing nearly every aspect of daily life. Here's a comprehensive look at why sleep is so important and how it impacts various aspects of health:

1. Physical Health

a. Immune System Function

- **Benefits**: Adequate sleep strengthens the immune system, helping the body fight off infections and illnesses.
- **Impact**: Chronic sleep deprivation can impair immune response, increasing susceptibility to diseases.

b. Cardiovascular Health

- **Benefits**: Quality sleep supports heart health by regulating blood pressure and reducing the risk of cardiovascular diseases.
- **Impact**: Poor sleep can contribute to high blood pressure, heart disease, and stroke.

c. Weight Management

- **Benefits**: Sleep regulates hormones that control hunger and appetite, aiding in weight management.
- **Impact**: Sleep deprivation can lead to weight gain by disrupting hunger signals and increasing cravings for high-calorie foods.

d. Hormone Regulation

- **Benefits**: Sleep helps regulate hormones that affect growth, stress, and metabolism.
- **Impact**: Inadequate sleep can disrupt hormone balance, leading to issues such as increased stress levels and impaired growth.

e. Muscle Repair and Growth

- **Benefits**: During deep sleep, the body repairs and builds muscle tissue.

- **Impact**: Insufficient sleep can hinder muscle recovery and growth, affecting physical performance.

2. Mental Health

a. Cognitive Function

- **Benefits**: Sleep is crucial for cognitive processes such as memory, attention, and problem-solving.
- **Impact**: Lack of sleep impairs cognitive function, leading to difficulties with concentration, decision-making, and learning.

b. Emotional Regulation

- **Benefits**: Quality sleep supports emotional stability and resilience.
- **Impact**: Sleep deprivation can lead to mood swings, irritability, and increased risk of mental health issues such as depression and anxiety.

c. Stress Management

- **Benefits**: Adequate sleep helps regulate stress levels and supports the body's ability to cope with stress.
- **Impact**: Poor sleep can exacerbate stress, making it more challenging to manage daily stressors.

3. Behavioral Health

a. Productivity and Performance

- **Benefits**: Well-rested individuals tend to be more productive, focused, and efficient in their daily tasks.
- **Impact**: Sleep deprivation can lead to decreased productivity, increased errors, and impaired job performance.

b. Safety

- **Benefits**: Adequate sleep improves alertness and reaction times, reducing the risk of accidents and injuries.
- **Impact**: Sleep deprivation increases the likelihood of accidents, both at home and on the road, due to impaired coordination and judgment.

c. Relationship Quality

- **Benefits**: Good sleep contributes to positive interactions and effective communication with others.

- **Impact**: Poor sleep can lead to conflicts and misunderstandings in personal and professional relationships due to irritability and decreased patience.

4. Sleep Stages and Their Functions

a. REM Sleep (Rapid Eye Movement)

- **Functions**: Essential for dreaming, memory consolidation, and emotional regulation.
- **Impact**: Insufficient REM sleep can affect memory retention and emotional stability.

b. Deep Sleep (Slow-Wave Sleep)

- **Functions**: Crucial for physical restoration, muscle repair, and growth.
- **Impact**: Lack of deep sleep can impair physical recovery and overall health.

c. Light Sleep

- **Functions**: Acts as a transitional phase between wakefulness and deep sleep, contributing to overall restfulness.
- **Impact**: Disruptions in light sleep can affect the quality of overall sleep.

5. Strategies for Improving Sleep Quality

a. Maintain a Consistent Sleep Schedule

- **Recommendations**: Go to bed and wake up at the same time every day, even on weekends, to regulate your body's internal clock.

b. Create a Relaxing Bedtime Routine

- **Recommendations**: Develop a calming pre-sleep routine, such as reading, taking a warm bath, or practicing relaxation techniques.

c. Optimize Sleep Environment

- **Recommendations**: Ensure a comfortable sleep environment with a supportive mattress, appropriate room temperature, and minimal noise and light.

d. Limit Exposure to Screens Before Bed

- **Recommendations**: Avoid screens (phones, tablets, computers) at least an hour before bedtime to reduce blue light exposure, which can interfere with sleep.

e. Manage Stress and Anxiety

- **Recommendations**: Practice stress-reducing techniques such as mindfulness, meditation, and deep breathing to promote relaxation before bed.

f. Avoid Caffeine and Heavy Meals Before Bed

- **Recommendations**: Limit caffeine intake in the afternoon and evening and avoid heavy or spicy meals close to bedtime to prevent sleep disturbances.

Conclusion

Sleep is essential for maintaining physical, mental, and emotional health. It supports immune function, cardiovascular health, hormone regulation, cognitive function, and emotional stability. Prioritizing good sleep hygiene and addressing factors that affect sleep quality can lead to significant improvements in overall well-being and quality of life. If sleep problems persist, consider seeking advice from a healthcare professional to identify and address any underlying issues.

Detoxification and Cleansing

Safe Detox Practices

Detoxification can be beneficial for overall health, but it's essential to approach it in a safe and effective manner to avoid potential risks and complications. Here are key principles and practices for ensuring a safe detox experience:

1. Understand Your Body's Needs

a. Assess Health Conditions

- **Considerations**: Consult with a healthcare professional if you have existing health conditions or are taking medications. Some detox methods may not be suitable for individuals with certain medical conditions.

b. Personalization

- **Guidelines**: Tailor detox practices to your individual needs and health status. What works for one person may not be appropriate for another.

2. Gradual and Balanced Approach

a. Avoid Extreme Detox Diets

- **Risks**: Extreme diets or fasting can lead to nutrient deficiencies, dehydration, and electrolyte imbalances.
- **Recommendations**: Opt for gradual changes, such as incorporating more fruits and vegetables into your diet, rather than extreme detox protocols.

b. Balanced Nutrition

- **Guidelines**: Ensure your detox plan includes a variety of nutrients to support overall health. Focus on whole foods like fruits, vegetables, whole grains, and lean proteins.

3. Stay Hydrated

a. Drink Plenty of Water

- **Benefits**: Adequate hydration supports kidney function and helps flush out toxins.
- **Recommendations**: Aim for at least 8 glasses of water per day. Herbal teas and infused water can also contribute to hydration.

b. Avoid Excessive Caffeine and Alcohol

- **Risks**: Both caffeine and alcohol can contribute to dehydration and may counteract detox efforts.
- **Guidelines**: Limit intake and focus on hydrating beverages.

4. Incorporate Gentle Detox Methods

a. Herbal Teas and Supplements

- **Examples**: Herbal teas like dandelion root, milk thistle, and green tea can support detoxification.
- **Recommendations**: Use supplements with guidance from a healthcare provider to avoid interactions or adverse effects.

b. Light Exercise

- **Benefits**: Regular physical activity promotes circulation and supports detoxification through sweating.
- **Recommendations**: Engage in moderate exercise such as walking, swimming, or yoga.

5. Monitor Your Body's Response

a. Pay Attention to Symptoms

- **Guidelines**: Monitor how your body responds to detox practices. Symptoms like fatigue, dizziness, or digestive discomfort may indicate that adjustments are needed.

b. Adjust as Needed

- **Recommendations**: If you experience adverse effects, modify your detox plan or consult with a healthcare professional for guidance.

6. Avoid Unsafe Practices

a. Extreme Fasting

- **Risks**: Extended fasting can lead to severe nutrient deficiencies, dehydration, and other health issues.
- **Recommendations**: Opt for shorter, less restrictive fasting methods or intermittent fasting, and always consult with a healthcare provider first.

b. Unsafe Cleansing Products

- **Risks**: Some over-the-counter detox products or cleanses can be harsh on the body and may cause side effects.
- **Guidelines**: Research and choose reputable products, and consider natural methods like dietary changes and hydration.

7. Focus on Long-Term Lifestyle Changes

a. Sustainable Practices

- **Benefits**: Incorporate detox-supportive habits into your daily routine for lasting benefits.
- **Recommendations**: Maintain a balanced diet, regular exercise, and adequate hydration as ongoing practices.

b. Stress Management

- **Techniques**: Include practices like meditation, mindfulness, and relaxation exercises to support overall health and well-being.

8. Consult with Healthcare Professionals

a. Seek Expert Advice

- **Guidelines**: Before starting any new detox regimen, especially if you have health conditions or are on medication, consult with a healthcare provider.

b. Regular Check-Ins

- **Recommendations**: Schedule regular check-ins with your healthcare provider to monitor progress and ensure safety.

Conclusion

Safe detox practices involve understanding your body's needs, adopting gradual and balanced approaches, staying hydrated, incorporating gentle methods, and avoiding extreme or unsafe practices. Monitoring your body's response and making necessary adjustments are crucial for ensuring a successful and healthy detox experience. Always seek guidance from healthcare professionals to tailor detox practices to your individual health needs and goals.

Daily Detox Tips

Incorporating detoxification practices into your daily routine can support overall health and well-being. Here are practical tips for daily detoxification:

1. Start Your Day with Water

a. Hydration Boost

- **Benefits**: Drinking a glass of water first thing in the morning helps kick-start your metabolism and flush out toxins that have accumulated overnight.
- **Tips**: Consider adding a squeeze of lemon for added detox benefits and a boost of Vitamin C.

2. Eat a Balanced Breakfast

a. Nutrient-Rich Foods

- **Benefits**: A balanced breakfast provides essential nutrients and helps regulate blood sugar levels.
- **Recommendations**: Include fruits, whole grains, and lean proteins. Options like oatmeal with berries or a smoothie with spinach and flaxseed are great choices.

3. Incorporate Detoxifying Foods

a. Include Cruciferous Vegetables

- **Benefits**: Vegetables like broccoli, kale, and Brussels sprouts support liver detoxification.
- **Tips**: Add these vegetables to salads, stir-fries, or soups.

b. Add Fiber-Rich Foods

- **Benefits**: Fiber supports digestive health and helps eliminate waste from the body.
- **Recommendations**: Consume foods like chia seeds, flaxseeds, and whole grains.

4. Stay Hydrated Throughout the Day

a. Regular Water Intake

- **Benefits**: Maintaining hydration supports kidney function and detoxification.
- **Recommendations**: Carry a reusable water bottle and aim for at least 8 glasses of water daily. Herbal teas can also contribute to hydration.

5. Move Your Body

a. Exercise Regularly

- **Benefits**: Physical activity boosts circulation and supports detoxification through sweating.
- **Recommendations**: Engage in at least 30 minutes of moderate exercise most days, such as walking, jogging, or yoga.

b. Incorporate Movement Breaks

- **Tips**: If you have a sedentary job, take short breaks to stretch or walk to keep your body active and support overall health.

6. Practice Deep Breathing

a. Stress Reduction

- **Benefits**: Deep breathing exercises help reduce stress and support lung function, aiding in the elimination of toxins through breath.
- **Recommendations**: Practice deep breathing or mindfulness for a few minutes each day.

7. Consume Herbal Teas

a. Detoxifying Herbs

- **Benefits**: Herbal teas such as dandelion root, green tea, and ginger can support liver function and overall detoxification.
- **Recommendations**: Enjoy a cup of herbal tea in the morning or afternoon for added detox benefits.

8. Avoid Processed Foods

a. Reduce Toxin Intake

- **Benefits**: Processed foods can contain additives and preservatives that may burden your detoxification systems.
- **Recommendations**: Focus on whole, unprocessed foods for better health and detoxification.

9. Practice Good Sleep Hygiene

a. Quality Sleep

- **Benefits**: Proper sleep supports the body's natural detoxification processes and overall health.
- **Recommendations**: Aim for 7-9 hours of quality sleep each night, and maintain a consistent sleep schedule.

10. Engage in Relaxation Techniques

a. Stress Management

- **Benefits**: Relaxation techniques help manage stress, which can impact detoxification.
- **Recommendations**: Practice techniques such as meditation, yoga, or gentle stretching to support mental and physical well-being.

11. Include Probiotics

a. Gut Health

- **Benefits**: Probiotics support a healthy gut microbiome, which is essential for digestion and detoxification.

- **Recommendations**: Include probiotic-rich foods like yogurt, kefir, or fermented vegetables in your diet.

12. Use Natural Skincare Products

a. Skin Health

- **Benefits**: Using natural skincare products reduces exposure to potentially harmful chemicals that can affect the body's detoxification processes.
- **Recommendations**: Opt for products with natural ingredients and avoid those with synthetic additives.

Conclusion

Daily detox tips involve simple yet effective practices that support the body's natural detoxification processes and promote overall health. By staying hydrated, eating a balanced diet, incorporating physical activity, managing stress, and using natural products, you can enhance your well-being and support your body's natural ability to detoxify. Consistency in these daily habits contributes to long-term health and vitality.

Mind-Body Connection

The Role of Mindfulness and Meditation

Mindfulness and meditation are powerful practices that play a significant role in enhancing mental and physical health. They help foster a deep connection between mind and body, reduce stress, and improve overall well-being. Here's an overview of their roles and benefits:

1. Understanding Mindfulness and Meditation

a. What is Mindfulness?

- **Definition**: Mindfulness involves being fully present and aware of the current moment without judgment. It means paying attention to thoughts, feelings, and sensations as they occur.
- **Practices**: Mindfulness can be practiced through various activities, including mindful eating, walking, and breathing.

b. What is Meditation?

- **Definition**: Meditation is a practice where an individual uses techniques like focused attention or guided imagery to achieve a state of mental clarity, relaxation, and insight.
- **Types**: Common forms include mindfulness meditation, loving-kindness meditation, and transcendental meditation.

2. Benefits of Mindfulness and Meditation

a. Stress Reduction

- **Impact**: Both mindfulness and meditation can significantly reduce stress by calming the mind and promoting relaxation.
- **Mechanism**: They help lower cortisol levels and activate the parasympathetic nervous system, which counteracts the stress response.

b. Improved Mental Clarity and Focus

- **Benefits**: Regular practice enhances concentration, attention span, and cognitive function.
- **Techniques**: Meditation practices like focusing on the breath or a mantra improve cognitive control and mental clarity.

c. Emotional Regulation

- **Effects**: Mindfulness and meditation help manage emotions by increasing awareness and acceptance of emotional states.
- **Outcomes**: They can lead to improved mood, reduced anxiety, and enhanced emotional resilience.

d. Better Sleep Quality

- **Benefits**: Practices that promote relaxation and reduce stress can improve sleep quality and help manage insomnia.
- **Recommendations**: Incorporate mindfulness or meditation into your bedtime routine for better sleep.

e. Enhanced Self-Awareness

- **Impact**: Mindfulness fosters greater self-awareness by encouraging reflection on thoughts, behaviors, and emotions.
- **Results**: Increased self-awareness can lead to more intentional living and improved decision-making.

f. Physical Health Benefits

- **Effects**: Regular practice has been linked to lower blood pressure, improved immune function, and reduced chronic pain.
- **Mechanism**: The stress-reducing effects of mindfulness and meditation contribute to overall physical health.

3. How to Practice Mindfulness

a. Mindful Breathing

- **Technique**: Focus on your breath, observing each inhale and exhale without altering your breathing pattern.
- **Practice**: Spend a few minutes each day practicing mindful breathing to cultivate a sense of calm.

b. Mindful Eating

- **Technique**: Pay full attention to the taste, texture, and aroma of your food, eating slowly and savoring each bite.
- **Benefits**: This practice enhances digestion and promotes a healthier relationship with food.

c. Mindful Walking

- **Technique**: Walk slowly and attentively, paying attention to the sensations in your feet, legs, and the surrounding environment.
- **Benefits**: Mindful walking can be a grounding practice that enhances awareness and relaxation.

4. How to Practice Meditation

a. Choose a Comfortable Position

- **Options**: Sit or lie down in a comfortable position that allows you to relax without discomfort.
- **Recommendations**: Use a cushion or chair if needed to support proper posture.

b. Focus on Your Breath or a Mantra

- **Breath Awareness**: Pay attention to your breathing, noting the sensation of each inhale and exhale.
- **Mantra Meditation**: Repeat a calming word or phrase silently to focus the mind and induce relaxation.

c. Start with Short Sessions

- **Duration**: Begin with 5-10 minutes of meditation and gradually increase the time as you become more comfortable with the practice.
- **Consistency**: Aim to practice daily or several times a week to build and maintain the benefits.

d. Use Guided Meditations

- **Resources**: Use apps, online videos, or audio recordings to guide you through meditation sessions, especially if you are new to the practice.
- **Benefits**: Guided meditations can provide structure and support, making it easier to stay focused.

5. Integrating Mindfulness and Meditation into Daily Life

a. Create a Routine

- **Suggestions**: Establish a regular time for mindfulness or meditation practice, such as in the morning or before bed.
- **Consistency**: Consistent practice enhances the long-term benefits of mindfulness and meditation.

b. Incorporate Mindfulness into Daily Activities

- **Examples**: Practice mindfulness during routine activities such as driving, showering, or washing dishes.
- **Approach**: Focus on the sensory experiences of these activities to stay present and engaged.

c. Seek Support and Resources

- **Options**: Join mindfulness or meditation groups, attend workshops, or use online resources to deepen your practice.
- **Community**: Connecting with others who practice mindfulness and meditation can provide motivation and support.

Conclusion

Mindfulness and meditation play crucial roles in enhancing mental and physical health. They offer benefits such as stress reduction, improved focus, emotional regulation, better sleep quality, and physical health improvements. By incorporating these practices into daily life, you can foster a greater mind-body connection and support overall well-being. Consistent practice, whether through mindfulness or meditation, can lead to lasting positive changes in your life.

Yoga and Stretching Exercises

Yoga and stretching exercises are integral components of a holistic wellness routine, offering numerous benefits for both physical and mental health. Here's a comprehensive guide to incorporating yoga and stretching into your wellness plan:

1. Benefits of Yoga and Stretching

a. Improved Flexibility

- **Effects**: Regular yoga and stretching increase flexibility by lengthening and relaxing muscles.
- **Benefits**: Enhanced flexibility can improve range of motion, reduce stiffness, and prevent injuries.

b. Enhanced Strength and Balance

- **Effects**: Many yoga poses build muscle strength and enhance balance through bodyweight resistance.
- **Benefits**: Improved strength and balance contribute to better posture and stability.

c. Stress Reduction and Relaxation

- **Effects**: Yoga and stretching promote relaxation by reducing muscle tension and calming the nervous system.
- **Benefits**: These practices can lower stress levels, improve mental clarity, and support emotional well-being.

d. Improved Posture

- **Effects**: Yoga and stretching help align the spine and strengthen postural muscles.
- **Benefits**: Better posture reduces strain on the back and neck, alleviating discomfort and promoting overall health.

e. Enhanced Circulation

- **Effects**: Stretching and yoga improve blood flow by promoting vascular health and reducing muscle tightness.
- **Benefits**: Enhanced circulation supports nutrient delivery to tissues and aids in recovery and healing.

f. Pain Relief

- **Effects**: Gentle stretching and yoga can relieve chronic pain conditions, such as lower back pain, by releasing muscle tension and improving mobility.
- **Benefits**: These practices can serve as complementary therapies for pain management.

2. Essential Yoga Poses

a. Mountain Pose (Tadasana)

- **Benefits**: Improves posture, balance, and alignment.
- **Instructions**: Stand with feet together, weight evenly distributed. Engage the thighs, lengthen the spine, and reach the arms overhead. Hold for 30 seconds to 1 minute.

b. Downward-Facing Dog (Adho Mukha Svanasana)

- **Benefits**: Stretches the hamstrings, calves, and spine; strengthens the arms and shoulders.
- **Instructions**: From a hands-and-knees position, lift the hips up and back, forming an inverted V. Press the heels towards the ground and hold for 30 seconds to 1 minute.

c. Warrior II (Virabhadrasana II)

- **Benefits**: Strengthens the legs, opens the hips, and improves balance.

- **Instructions**: Step one foot back, bend the front knee, and extend the arms out to the sides. Gaze over the front hand and hold for 30 seconds to 1 minute on each side.

d. Child's Pose (Balasana)

- **Benefits**: Gently stretches the back, hips, and thighs; promotes relaxation.
- **Instructions**: Kneel on the mat, sit back on your heels, and extend the arms forward, lowering the forehead to the floor. Hold for 1 to 2 minutes.

e. Cat-Cow Pose (Marjaryasana-Bitilasana)

- **Benefits**: Increases spine flexibility, stretches the back, and helps relieve lower back tension.
- **Instructions**: On hands and knees, alternate between arching the back (cat) and dipping it (cow), coordinating with your breath. Repeat for 1 to 2 minutes.

3. Effective Stretching Exercises

a. Hamstring Stretch

- **Benefits**: Stretches the hamstrings and lower back.
- **Instructions**: Sit on the floor with one leg extended and the other bent. Reach towards the extended leg, keeping the back straight. Hold for 20-30 seconds on each side.

b. Hip Flexor Stretch

- **Benefits**: Stretches the hip flexors and quads.
- **Instructions**: Step one foot forward into a lunge position, keeping the back leg straight. Push the hips forward gently and hold for 20-30 seconds on each side.

c. Shoulder Stretch

- **Benefits**: Stretches the shoulders and upper back.
- **Instructions**: Bring one arm across the chest and use the opposite arm to gently pull it closer to the body. Hold for 20-30 seconds on each side.

d. Side Stretch

- **Benefits**: Stretches the side body, including the obliques and lats.
- **Instructions**: Stand with feet hip-width apart, raise one arm overhead, and lean to the opposite side. Hold for 20-30 seconds on each side.

e. Upper Back Stretch

- **Benefits**: Stretches the upper back and between the shoulder blades.

- **Instructions**: Clasp your hands in front of you, round the upper back, and push the hands away from the body. Hold for 20-30 seconds.

4. Creating a Yoga and Stretching Routine

a. Set Realistic Goals

- **Suggestions**: Determine your objectives, such as improving flexibility, reducing stress, or relieving pain, and tailor your practice accordingly.

b. Establish a Consistent Schedule

- **Recommendations**: Aim to practice yoga or stretching 2-3 times a week, gradually increasing frequency as desired.

c. Warm Up Before Practice

- **Benefits**: Warming up prepares the muscles and reduces the risk of injury.
- **Suggestions**: Start with light cardio or dynamic stretches to increase circulation before yoga or static stretching.

d. Cool Down After Practice

- **Benefits**: Cooling down helps relax the muscles and promotes recovery.
- **Suggestions**: Incorporate gentle stretches or relaxation poses, such as Child's Pose, at the end of your routine.

e. Listen to Your Body

- **Advice**: Pay attention to your body's signals and avoid pushing beyond your limits. Modify poses and stretches as needed to accommodate your level of flexibility and strength.

f. Use Props if Needed

- **Options**: Utilize yoga blocks, straps, or bolsters to support your practice and enhance alignment.

5. Resources and Guidance

a. Yoga Classes and Online Resources

- **Options**: Consider joining a local yoga class or using online platforms for guided sessions and tutorials.
- **Benefits**: Access to experienced instructors and structured classes can help deepen your practice and ensure proper technique.

b. Stretching Apps and Videos

- **Suggestions**: Use apps or online videos that provide stretching routines and guidance for various fitness levels and goals.

c. Consult a Professional

- **Advice**: If you have specific health conditions or concerns, consult a healthcare professional or certified yoga instructor for personalized recommendations and modifications.

Conclusion

Yoga and stretching exercises are valuable practices for enhancing flexibility, strength, balance, and relaxation. By incorporating these practices into your routine, you can support overall well-being, improve posture, and manage stress. Create a balanced routine that includes a variety of poses and stretches, and seek guidance from resources or professionals to optimize your practice.

Emotional Wellness

Emotional wellness is a key component of overall well-being, encompassing the ability to understand, manage, and express emotions in a healthy and constructive way. It involves maintaining a balanced emotional state, developing resilience, and fostering positive relationships. Here's a comprehensive guide to enhancing and maintaining emotional wellness:

1. Understanding Emotional Wellness

a. What is Emotional Wellness?

- **Definition**: Emotional wellness refers to the state of being in which individuals effectively manage their emotions, cope with stress, and maintain a positive outlook on life. It includes understanding and expressing emotions appropriately, maintaining healthy relationships, and dealing with challenges constructively.

b. Components of Emotional Wellness

- **Self-Awareness**: Recognizing and understanding your own emotions and their impact on your behavior.
- **Self-Regulation**: Managing and controlling emotional responses, especially in stressful situations.
- **Resilience**: The ability to recover from setbacks and adapt to change.
- **Social Support**: Building and maintaining healthy relationships and seeking support when needed.

2. Strategies for Enhancing Emotional Wellness

a. Self-Awareness and Reflection

- **Practice Mindfulness**: Engage in mindfulness practices to become more aware of your emotions and reactions. This can involve meditation, deep breathing, or simply paying attention to your thoughts and feelings.
- **Journaling**: Write about your experiences, emotions, and reflections. Journaling can help you process and understand your feelings more deeply.

b. Emotional Regulation Techniques

- **Cognitive Behavioral Techniques**: Challenge and reframe negative thought patterns to alter emotional responses. Techniques such as identifying cognitive distortions and practicing positive self-talk can be beneficial.
- **Stress Management**: Incorporate stress-relief techniques such as deep breathing, progressive muscle relaxation, or engaging in hobbies to manage emotional responses effectively.

c. Building Resilience

- **Develop a Growth Mindset**: Embrace challenges as opportunities for growth and learning. Focus on solutions and adapt to changing circumstances.
- **Set Realistic Goals**: Break down goals into manageable steps and celebrate achievements. Setting and achieving goals can build confidence and resilience.
- **Practice Gratitude**: Regularly acknowledge and appreciate positive aspects of your life. Keeping a gratitude journal or expressing thanks to others can improve emotional well-being.

d. Fostering Positive Relationships

- **Effective Communication**: Practice open and honest communication with others. Active listening, empathy, and assertiveness contribute to healthy relationships.
- **Build a Support Network**: Cultivate relationships with supportive friends, family, and colleagues. Having a network of people you can rely on enhances emotional stability and provides a sense of belonging.

e. Seeking Professional Support

- **Therapy and Counseling**: Professional support from a therapist or counselor can provide tools and strategies for managing emotions, resolving conflicts, and addressing mental health concerns.
- **Support Groups**: Join support groups related to specific issues or experiences. Sharing experiences and learning from others can provide comfort and insights.

3. Practices to Support Emotional Wellness

a. Self-Care Routine

- **Physical Self-Care**: Engage in activities that promote physical health, such as regular exercise, adequate sleep, and healthy eating. Physical well-being is closely linked to emotional wellness.
- **Mental and Emotional Self-Care**: Schedule time for activities that bring joy and relaxation, such as reading, hobbies, or spending time with loved ones.

b. Healthy Boundaries

- **Identify Limits**: Recognize your limits and set boundaries to protect your emotional health. Learn to say no when necessary and prioritize self-care.
- **Respect Others' Boundaries**: Understand and respect the boundaries of others to maintain healthy and respectful relationships.

c. Emotional Expression

- **Creative Outlets**: Use creative activities such as art, music, or writing to express and process emotions.
- **Physical Activity**: Engage in physical activities that help release built-up emotions and improve mood.

d. Problem-Solving Skills

- **Develop Solutions**: Approach challenges with a problem-solving mindset. Break down problems into manageable parts and seek solutions actively.
- **Seek Feedback**: Discuss issues with trusted individuals and seek constructive feedback to gain new perspectives and solutions.

4. Addressing Common Emotional Challenges

a. Anxiety and Stress

- **Techniques**: Practice relaxation techniques, such as meditation or deep breathing, to manage anxiety. Consider mindfulness practices and seek support if needed.
- **Lifestyle Changes**: Incorporate stress-reducing activities into your routine, such as exercise, balanced nutrition, and adequate rest.

b. Depression

- **Recognize Symptoms**: Be aware of signs of depression, such as persistent sadness, loss of interest, or changes in sleep and appetite.
- **Seek Help**: If experiencing symptoms of depression, consult a mental health professional for appropriate treatment and support.

c. Relationship Issues

- **Communication Skills**: Work on improving communication skills and addressing conflicts constructively. Seek couples or family therapy if needed.
- **Self-Reflection**: Reflect on your role in relationship dynamics and make efforts to improve interactions and understanding.

Conclusion

Emotional wellness is crucial for overall well-being and involves managing emotions, building resilience, and fostering positive relationships. By practicing self-awareness, emotional regulation, and self-care, you can enhance your emotional health and cope effectively with life's challenges. Seek professional support when needed and build a supportive network to maintain and improve your emotional wellness.

Conclusion

In closing, achieving and maintaining optimal wellness involves a holistic approach that encompasses physical, emotional, mental, and spiritual health. Each component of wellness interconnects and influences the others, creating a comprehensive and balanced approach to well-being. Here's a summary of key takeaways from this book:

1. Embrace a Holistic Perspective

- **Integration**: Recognize that wellness is not just about treating symptoms but addressing underlying causes and fostering overall balance in life. Integrate various aspects of health—nutrition, exercise, emotional well-being, and mindfulness—to create a harmonious lifestyle.

- **Personalization**: Tailor your wellness plan to suit your unique needs and preferences. What works for one person might not be ideal for another, so customize protocols, practices, and routines to fit your individual goals and circumstances.

2. Incorporate Effective Practices

- **Herbal Protocols**: Utilize herbal remedies and natural therapies to support health and address common ailments. Follow guidelines for safe and effective use, and consult with healthcare professionals if needed.

- **Nutrition and Exercise**: Adopt a balanced diet and regular exercise routine that aligns with your health goals. Emphasize whole foods, mindful eating, and appropriate physical activities to enhance overall wellness.

- **Emotional Wellness**: Prioritize emotional health through self-awareness, stress management, and positive relationships. Practice mindfulness, seek professional support when needed, and engage in activities that promote emotional resilience and satisfaction.

3. Foster Healthy Habits and Routines

- **Consistency**: Build and maintain healthy habits by incorporating wellness practices into your daily routine. Consistent efforts contribute to long-term benefits and overall well-being.

- **Adaptability**: Be open to adapting your wellness plan as your needs and circumstances change. Flexibility allows you to address new challenges and opportunities for growth effectively.

4. Seek Support and Resources

- **Professional Guidance**: Don't hesitate to seek advice from healthcare professionals, nutritionists, or wellness coaches to optimize your health journey. Their expertise can provide valuable insights and personalized recommendations.

- **Community and Resources**: Connect with support groups, wellness communities, and educational resources to gain additional support, knowledge, and motivation.

5. Celebrate Progress and Achievements

- **Acknowledgment**: Recognize and celebrate your achievements and progress towards your wellness goals. Celebrating milestones, no matter how small, reinforces positive behaviors and motivates continued efforts.

- **Gratitude**: Cultivate a sense of gratitude for the improvements and positive changes in your life. Acknowledging and appreciating your efforts enhances overall well-being and satisfaction.

Final Thoughts

Your journey to holistic wellness is a dynamic and ongoing process. By embracing a comprehensive approach that includes physical, emotional, and mental health practices, you can create a balanced and fulfilling life. Remember that wellness is not a destination but a continuous journey of growth and self-care. Embrace each step of the journey with openness, curiosity, and commitment, and enjoy the benefits of a healthier, more vibrant life.

Made in the USA
Middletown, DE
29 August 2024